Miracles of MOTHER TINCTURES

with
Therapeutic Hints
and
Treatment of Diseases

by
DR. YADUBIR SINHA, M.D.S. (U.S.A.)
Ex-Principal, The Sinha Homoeopathic Medical College
and Hospital (Govt. Affiliated, Recognised and Aided)
P.O. Laheriasarai (Bihar)

B. Jain Publishers (P) Ltd.
USA—EUROPE—INDIA

MIRACLES OF MOTHER TINCTURES WITH THERAPEUTIC HINTS AND TREATMENT OF DISEASES

34th Impression 2024

All rights reserved. No part of this book may be reproduced, stored in a retrieval system or transmitted, in any form or by any means, mechanical, photocopying, recording or otherwise, without any prior written permission of the publisher.

© with the publisher

Published by Kuldeep Jain for
B. JAIN PUBLISHERS (P) LTD.
B. Jain House, D-157, Sector-63,
NOIDA-201307, U.P. (INDIA)
Tel.: +91-120-4933333 • *Email:* info@bjain.com
Website: **www.bjain.com**

Printed in India

ISBN: 978-81-319-0098-7

PUBLISHER'S NOTE

This book is an outcome of a learned author's untiresome labour of many year's research, experiments and experience, with the Homeopathic Mother Tincture Therapy. The author has given the therapeutic application of these remedies which were organised by Master Hahnemann from the western sources, and has also included a wide range of those plants and herbs which are easily available in India and are having the infallible curative properties in their tincture form. The miraculous action of these Mother Tinctures as depicted by Dr. Yadubir Sinha can, no doubt be applied to heal in many conditions said to be 'incurable' by the other systems of medicine.

With this hope that the work may be easily available to thousands of our patron homeopaths all over the globe and it may prove a boon to whole of the ailing race, we have come forward to publish this present revised edition. However, we shall still remain indebted to our patrons if they could point out the mistakes, if any, of the present edition of being rectified in the next edition.

10th April, 1981 **Kuldeep Jain**
C.E.O., B. Jain Publishers (P) Ltd.

INTRODUCTION

This unique book of its type has been written with great endeavour and sincerity with the purpose of acquainting our homoeopathic practitioners with infallible drugs. This book contains the most valuable prescriptions and experiences of the world renowned homoeopathic physicians who have gained laurels by dint of using these Mother Tinctures.

In the hurry and bustle of the age, the physician is not in a position to devote much time to reach the similimum. Allopathy-minded patients demand immediate relief of ailments. For this end in view, this book is indeed a marvellous one. Many of the Mother Tinctures will at once arrest the progress of the disease and afford instant cure where only prompt relief can be obtained in some cases where chronic miasms have their root deep in the cells. In such cases relief should be given and then attempt should be made for radical cure by application of the most similar drugs of high potency.

If this book-let proves to be beneficial to the patients and practitioners, I am amply rewarded.

10th April, 1962 **The Author**

CONTENTS
CHAPTER

Diseases	*Pages*
Abortion	1
Amenorrhoea	1
Asthma	2
Acne	2
Anaemia	2
Apoplexy	2
Bleeding from Piles	3
Bleeding from Lungs	3
Beri-beri (Droptical Effusion in Lower Extremities, Weakness etc.)	3
Bubo	3
Cholera	4
Chlorosis	4
Coryza	4
Collapse	4
Chorea	5
Cough	5
Constipation	5
Diarrhoea	6
Dysentery	6
Dysmenorrhoea	6
Diphtheria	6
Dyspepsia	7
Dropsy	7

Diseases	Pages
Enlargement of Liver	7
Epilepsy	8
Elephantiasis	9
Enlargement of Spleen	9
Enlargement of Uterus	9
Gall-stones and Biliary Colics	9
Goitre	10
Gonorrhoea	10
Hydrophobia	11
Haemorrhagic Dysentery	11
Haemorrhage	11
Hysteria	12
Hiccough	12
Heart Affections	12
High Blood Pressure	12
Insomnia	13
Insanity	13
Impotency	13
Intermittent Fever	13
Jaundice	13
Kalaazar	13
Leprosy	14
Labour Pains	14
Leucorrhoea	14
Menstrual Disorder	15
Mental Weakness	15
Neuralgia	15
Nocturnal Emissions	15
Nervous Debility	16
Night Blindness	16

Diseases	Pages
Obesity	16
Phthisis	16
Puerperal Fever	18
Paralysis	18
Pits of Pox	18
Palpitation of Heart	18
Rheumatism and Gout	18
Snake Bite	19
Septi Caemia	19
Suppression of Urine	19
Spermatorrhoea	29
Suppression of Milk	20
Senselessness	20
Skin Diseases	20
Spasms	21
Syphilis	21
Tremour	21
Tetanus	22
Tumour	22
Uterine Disorder	22

CHAPTER II (A)

Remedies

Abroma Augusta	24
Abroma Radix	24
Abrotanum	25
Acalypha Indica	26
Aeglefolia Bilwapatra	26
Aegla Marmelos	27
Aconite Radix	27

Remedies	Pages
Aconite Nap	27
Acenasia	28
Acid Hydro	28
Arsenic Alb	29
Anacardium	29
Aloes	29
Apocynum	29
Agaricus	29
Aletris of Farinosa	30
Amyl Nitric	31
Arnithogallum Ambeletum	31
Alfalfa	31
Avena Sativa	32
Asoka Janosia	34
Arjun Terminalia Arjnua	35
Atista Indica Q	35
Atista Radix	36
Asai	36
Azadirecta Indica	36
Andersonia Rohitak	37
Aswagandha	37
Alstonia Scholaris	38
Asparagus Officinalis	38
Absinthium	39
Adonis Vernalis	39
Agave Americana	39
Alunus	40
Ambrosia	40
Amygdatus Persica	40

Remedies	Pages
Apocynum Androsacimic Folium	40
Apomorphia	41
Agnilegia	41
Aralia Racemosa	41
Arania Diodema	42
Arbutus Andraohev	42
Arsenic Bromatum	43
Asclepias Syriaca	43
Aspid Osperma	43
Aurum Mur Natronatum	43
Asarum Europium	44
Amalki	44
Aqua Ptychosis	44
Achyranthus Asperolin	44
Baryta Iod	45
Beta Vulgaris	45
Betonica	45
Boletus Taricis	45
Blata Orientalis	46
Blumia Odorata	47
Boerrhavia Diffusa	47
Borrhavia Repense	47
Berberis Aquifolia	47
Bryophyllum Calycinum	48
Bufo Rana	48
Berberis Vulgaris	49
Bellis Perennis	49
Baptisia	50
Belladonna	50

Remedies	Pages
Caladium Seguinum	50
Camphor	51
Carduus Marianus	51
Cascara Amarga	53
Ceanothus Americanus	53
Convallaria Majolis	54
Crataegus Oxyacantha	54
Cactus Grandifolius	55
Coccus Cacti	55
Chaparo Amargosa	55
Cenic Cio	55
Castor oil	55
Chirata	56
Coffea Mocha	56
Cubeb	56
Canabis Sativa	56
Canabis Indica	57
Croton Tig	57
Carica Papaya	57
Cantharis	57
Cimicifuga	58
Cod Liver Oil	58
Condurango	58
Cina	58
Chininum Sulph	59
Cedron	59
Chionanthus	59
Cholestrinum	60
Caffein	60

Remedies	*Pages*
Chimaphilla	65
Clematis	60
Cornus Acternifolia	61
Chloralum	61
Chlorate Hydrate	61
Crocus	61
Chomocladia	61
Crisophanic Acid	61
Ceasalpania Bondulosa	61
Calotropis Gigantia	62
Calotropis Uactum	63
Cleldendron Infortunata	63
Cephalendra Indica	63
Coleus Aromaticus	64
Cyndon Dactylone	64
Caulophyllum	65
Desmodium Gingeticum	66
Damiana	66
Dioscorea	67
Drosera	68
Dulcamara	69
Eupatorium	69
Eupatorium Ayapan	70
Euphorbium	70
Euphorbia Pilulifera	70
Euphrasia	70
Embelia Riebens	71
Echinacea Augustifolia	71
Esculentine	74
Euesl yptus Globe	75

Remedies	Pages
Equisetum	75
Ficcus Religiosa	75
Ficcus Indica	76
Ferrum Phos	76
Fluid Cerifolius	77
Fraximus Americana	77
Fucus Vesiculosus	78
Fluid Calendula	78
Geranium Maculatum	78
Gallium Aperine	79
Gelsemium	79
Glonoine	80
Grindalia	81
Guaiacum	82
Gynocardia Odorata **Chalmogra**	82
Hamamelis	82
Heleborus Niger	83
Helonias Dioica	84
Hydrastis	84
Hydrocotyle Asiatica	86
Hydrocyanic Acid	87
Hypericum	87
Hymosa	88
Helarrhena or Chenomorha **Anti-Dy**senterica Kurchi	89
Hygrophilla Spinosa	89
Hemidesmus Indica	90
Hydrophobin	90
Jacranda Caroba	90
Jatropha Curcas	91

Remedies	Pages
Justicia Adhatoda	91
Justicia Rubrum	92
Jaborandi	92
Kalmegh	92
Lufa Bindal	92
Lufa Amara or Fuetida	93
Leucus Aspera	93
Lauhyrus Sativus	94
Laurocerasus	94
Lobelia Inflata	94
Malaria Officinalis	97
Manganese Dioxide	98
Makaradhwaj	95
Menispernum	95
Mutha	95
Mica	95
Momordica Cherentia	96
Mullen Oil	96
Nyctanthus	96
Natrum MurBit	97
Nufer Leuteum	98
Nux Juglans	98
Nux Vomica	98
Oldenlandia Herbecea	98
Oenanthe Crocata	98
Ocimum Sanctum	99
Ova Testa	99
Origanum	99
Pas Avena	99
Passiflora Compound	100

Remedies	Pages
Passiflora Incarnata	100
Prerero Brena	101
Phytoline	101
Pulsatilla	102
Recinus Communis	102
Ranwolfia Serpentina	102
Ruta	103
Symphoricarpus Recemosa	103
Spiritus Glandium Quercus	103
Succus Amogara	103
Syzygium Jambolinum	103
Solanum Xanthocarpum	104
Secale Cor	104
Strophanthus	105
Symphytum	105
Saw Palenetto	105
Santonine	105
Stigmata Medius	106
Sebal Serrulata	106
Spongia	106
Salix Nigra	106
Senega	106
Strychnia Phos	107
Saracenia	107
Sulphur	107
Cimicio	107
Tinospora Cordifolia	107
Thymol	108
Tricosanthes Disica	108
Tribulus Terrestris	108

Remedies	Pages
Thlapsi Bursa Pastoris	109
Thyroidine	109
Trillium	109
Tathelin	109
Vesicaria Communis	109
Viburnum Opulus	110
Viburnum Prunifolium	110
Vaccininum Metallicum	111
Viscum Album	111
Valariana	111
Zincum Valariana	111

CHAPTER II (B)

External Mother Tinctures ... 112

CHAPTER III

Therapeutic Hints ... 121

CHAPTER I
TREATMENT OF DISEASES WITH MOTHER TINCTURES

1. Abortion

Haemorrhage from the womb in early months. Premature delivery of a dead child in later months is called miscarriage.

Blumia odorata 2, 1x—Bleeding from uterus in gushes during or after abortion when all other remedies have failed.

Cimicifuga Q—To ensure the birth of alive child in expectant mothers who are disappointed due to delivering of dead children. 5 drops thrice daily since fifth month.

Helonias Q—Abortion with excessive bleeding and sensation of presence of uterus with weak womb.

Trillium 1x—Specific remedy.

2. Amenorrhoea

Suppression of menses.

Asoka Q—Specific and intercurrent remedy in all cases.

Secale Q—Extremly hot patient, weak, thin with strong craving for cold and cold air.

Pulsatilla Q—Phlegmatic, hot women with mild disposition, open air and cold bathing ameliorates.

Sulphur Q—Heat general, weak subjects, aversion to bathing in winter, frequent baths in summer and open air hunger.

Do not misuse these medicines, or they will cause abortion and then will be controlled *by China, Ipecac, Ferrum phos* and anti-haemorrhagic medicines.

3. Asthma

Dyspnoea, difficulty in breathing associated with cardiac, bronchial or digestive affections.

Blatta orientalis Q—During paroxysm and 3x in the interval in corpulent subjects of malarial origin.

Passiflora incarnata Q—1 dr. in paroxysm, one dose.

Cannabis sativa Q—Can breathe only when standing.

Makaradhwaj Q—Specially when the heart is weak or affected.

See *Senega*.

4. Acne

Small pimples on face with or without pain.
Nux juglans Q—In young girls.

Kali brom 3x—General medicine.

5. Anaemia

Loss of blood with pale or waxy complexion of face.

Ferrum phos 2x—The specific remedy.

May be assisted by *Calc phos* and *Natrum mur* in chlorotic school girls.

6. Apoplexy

Rush of blood to the head with loss of consciousness and impairment of nerves.

Laurocerasus Q, 1x—Specific remedy.

7. Bleeding Piles

Discharge of blood during or after stool with or without pain etc.

Blumia odorata Q, *1x* – Specific remedy.

8. Bleeding from Lungs

Acalypha indica Q, *1x* – Haemorrhage of bright red blood in the morning and that of dark, clotted blood in the afternoon with incessant cough at night.

Ficcus religiosa Q, *1x* – Bright red blood from lungs.

Blumia odorata Q, *1x* – Pulmonary haemorrhage with dry, barking, sawing cough with wheezing sound, aphonia, hoarseness.

Hamamelis Q – Venous blood of dark colour.

Cyndon dactylon Q, *1x* – Alternate this with *Geranium mac* **Q** in all cases.

Justicia rubrum Q, *1x* – Bleeding from lungs with paroxysms of cough in pthisical subjects.

Occimum sanctum Q, *1x* – Phlegm, streaked with blood in early stage.

Eupatorium ayapan Q, *1x* – With cough in consumptives having haemorrhagic diathesis in history.

9. Beri-beri

Dropsical effusion in lower extremities, weakness etc.

Lathyrus Q, *1x* – To be alternated with *China* in all cases.

10. Bubo

Bufo rana Q, *1x* – Specific remedy.

11. Cholera

Violent vomiting purging, cramps, thirst and sudden prostration, suppression or retention of urine.

Camphor Q—In the beginning or collapse stage with internal burning, external coldness, dryness of skin, desires to be uncovered, sudden prostration.

Coffea mocha Q—10 drops every 10 minutes only three doses in all stages.

Recinus Q, 1x—Prominently of diarrhoeic type.

Trycho santhis Q, 1x—Nearly a specific in all stages.

12. Chlorosis

Loss of blood with blueness of face and veins etc.

Abroma augusta—With dysmenorrhoea, penis causing shrieks, constipation, profuse micturition and irritable temper.

Asoka Q—With menstrual disorder or leucorrhoea.

Carpus leuteum 1x—Specific in all cases.

13. Coryza

Cold.

Camphor Q—In the very beginning.

Occimum Q—Running of nose with cough.

14. Collapse

Last stage, pulse weak, imperceptible, cold body, etc.

Camphor Q—Revives heart and brain soon where indicated.

Hydrocyanic acid 2x—In gasping for breath, as if this is the last breath.

Aconite nap Q, 1x—Coldness of body, face cyanotic and like a corpse, great agony, restlessness, beats of heart regular with imperceptible pulse and fear of death.

Aconite radix 1x—Coldness and blueness of the whole body, respiration very difficult and cold, vertigo, pulse feeble, imperceptible.

Zinc cyanide 1x—When death is inevitable.

Caffein 1x—Use it in cases of heart failure.

15. Chorea

Dancing and jerking of muscles.

Pass Avena—Generally tones up nerves.

16. Cough

A concomitant symptom in many diseases.

Abroma aug 1x, 2—Cough with diabetes, constipation or dysmenorrhoea.

Cyndon dactylone 1x—With haemorrhage from lungs.

Justisia adhatoda—A general cough remedy. See *Justisia Rubrum*.

17. Constipation

Nonevacuation of stool due to inactivity or dryness of intestines and rectum.

Abroma augusta 1x—Hard, dry stools in diabetes.

Castor oil in one drop dose is a specific purgative.

Azadirecta indica Q, 1x—Constipation in chronic malaria.

Andersonia 1x—*Constipation* in malaria subjects.

18. Diarrhoea

A passing of loose watery stools.

Achyranthus asperalin 2, 1x — Frequent painless, watery profuse involuntary stools with vomiting, prostration, intense thirst retention of urine.

Camphor 2 — With coldness and collapse.

Chaparo amorgosa — Specific in most chronic cases.

Mutha 2 — Diarrhoea with indigestion.

19. Dysentery

Frequent stools of mucus and blood with tenesmus etc.

Alstonia 1x — Dysentery with diarrhoea specially in malaria patients.

Aegale marmelos Q, 1x — In the beginning stage.

Castor oil Q — One drop, to clear the bowels.

Cephalandra indica Q, 1x — Dysentery in malarial subjects.

Helarana anti-dysentria Q — It is worth its name.

20. Dysmenorrhoea

Painful scanty menstruation.

Abroma radix Q — Violent pain causing shrieks and shrills.

Xanthoxyllum Q, 1x — In all cases and as an alternative to **Abr**oma.

Ashoka — When the period is over, use it as an intercurrent remedy.

Cimicifuga Q, 1x — More the discharge more the pain increases with chronic uterine disorders in hysteric sensitive women.

21. Diphtheria

Thick membranes on tongue and inside throat with malignancy and stupor.

Echinacia Q, 1x—The specific remedy.

Acenasia Q, 1x—Great languor, cold sweat, fetid breath with or without haemorrhage of dark blood.

22. Dyspepsia

Indigestion, constipation, flatulence, loss of appetite or ravenous hunger.

Carica papaya 1x, trit.—Is regarded as a patent medicine.

Aqua phychota 1x—As an alternative remedy.

23. Dropsy

Aegle folioa Q—Dropsy with febrile conditions.

Borrhabia diffusa or ripens Q—In the beginning and *1x* in later stages is a well nigh specific.

Apocynum 1x—Dropsy with heart affections and menstrual troubles ; intense thirst but water disagrees in chilly patients

Convallaria majalis Q, 1x—Dropsy due to sluggish action of heart, dyspnoea, palpitation, scanty urine.

Lathyrus 1x—Specially in dropsy of beri-beri.

24. Enlargement of Liver

Liver enlarged with pain in it.

Azaredicta indica Q, 1x—Cases of suppressed malaria with **Quinine**.

Asia Q, 1x—Liver affections in last stage of **Kalaazar** when cerebral and cardiac affections predominate.

Andersonia Q, *1x*—Liver troubles of material origin with constipation with burning.

Carduus Q—Torpid liver, a specific remedy in all cases.

Quinia indica Q, *1x*—Intermittent fever with liver troubles.

Carica papaya Q, *1x*—When dyspepsia is a prominent affection.

Kalmegh Q, *1x*—Specific for an infantile liver and liver affections of **Kalaazar**.

Chlorodendron infortunata Q, *1x*—Liver enlarged with complaints of worm, diarrhoea and intermittent fever.

Lucus aspera Q, *1x*—Chronic malaria with enlarged liver, loss of appetite.

25. Epilepsy

Sudden fainting fits with the moon phases with foaming at mouth, lockjaw or convulsions with *aurra* starting from any place before falling into swoon.

Bufo rana Q, *1x*—Old adulterates having secret vices—a specific remedy.

Oenanthe crocata Q, *1x*—It is also an another specific remedy in all stages.

Hydrocyanic acid *2x*—Attended with difficult expiration and long gaping, contortions, convulsions, etc.

Veratrum viride *1x*—With rush of blood to head, pulse strong, red line in the middle of tongue.

Passavena Q—When nervous pains and irritation is prominent.

Passiflora inconata—To induce sleep and pacify cerebellum.

26. Elephantiasis

Thickening of feet like those of elephant due to filarial swelling.

Hydrocotyle asia Q, *1x* and *Anacardium 6*—Have been regarded as specifics in alternation.

27. Enlargement of Spleen

Ceanothus Q, *1x*—Internally and externally is a specific for enlarged spleen and splenitis.

Azaredicta Q, *Asai* Q, *Andersonia* Q, *Quinia Indica* Q, *Chlorodendron Infortunata,* Q and *Leupus aspera* Q—They do cure splenic affections if attended with malarial fever specially when suppressed by *quinine*.

Carica papya 1x—In dyspeptics.

Calotropis lactum—Specially in cases having presence or history of syphilitic poison.

Leupus aspera Q, *1x*—With loss of voice.

28. Enlargement of Uterus

Fraxinus americana Q, *1x*—It is specific for enlargement of uterus.

29. Gall Stones and Biliary Colics

Violent pain in hepatic region with bilious manifestations while stones are passing.

Carduus Q, *1x*—When liver is prominently affected with torpidity, constipation, etc.

Berberis Q, *1x*—When urinary symptoms are prominent, affections of left kidney, renal colic.

Chionanthus Q, *1x*—Associated with constant pain under right shoulder.

Dioscorea Q, 1x—When pain ameliorates on bending backward.

Cholestrinum 1x—Specific remedy to be used independently or in alternation with other remedies.

Stigmata madagus Q, 1x—Relieves at once the violent pain if given during poroxysm.

Parera Brava Q, 1x—Renal colic, difficult micturition with strong urging, fullness, violent pain in bladder and back, crying bitterly, red sand or brick dust in urine.

Thlapsi Bursa Pastoris Q, 1x—Renal colic with haematuria and dropsy.

Cactus Q, 1x—Gall stones or renal colic with constriction and cardiac affections.

30. Goitre

Enlargement of cervical glands in big size.

Iodine 1x—Internally and externally acts like a patent medicine.

Thyroiodine 1x—If goitre is attended with retarded physical and mental growth, emaciation etc.

Fucus vesiculosus Q, 1x—Goitre in subjects with obesity.

31. Gonorrhoea

Frequent painful, scanty urine with tenesmus and discharge of pus from urethra.

Cubeba Q, 1x—Thick yellow pus during micturition.

Vesicarea com. Q, 1x—Specific remedy in all cases.

Cannabis Sat Q, 1x—Patient walks with legs wide apart.

Coleus aromatics Q, 1x—With haematuria nephiritis or cystitis, discharge of mucus membrance, deposit of red sand.

32. Hydrophobia

Terrified at the sight of water or shining things after bite of mad dog or jackal.

Echinacea Q—Is a specific remedy.

33. Haemorrhagic Dysentery

Passing of huge amount of blood in dysentery.

Castor oil 1—In one drop dose to clear the bowels.

Atista radix Q, 1x—When emission of blood is prominent.

Cephalandra indica Q, 1x—Mucous and blood, green stools, with pain in navel region when all other remedies have failed.

Eupatorium ayapan Q, 1x—In haemorrhagic diathesis.

Baptisia 1x—When dysentery assumes a typhoid state with malignancy and prostration.

Vaccininum metallicum Q—Gangrneous stage of intestines; dysentery with foul blood.

Aloes Q, 1x—Muocus and blood with prolapsus ani and loss of power of sphincter nto resulting in involuntary discharges.

34. Haemorrhage

Passing of blood passive or active.

Cyndon dactylon Q, 1x—Haemorrhages from orifices.

Ficcus religiosa Q, 1x—Bright red blood from any orifice of body.

Hamamelis Q, 1x—Dark blood.

Ferrum phos 2x—Specially in bleeding after injury or with febrile conditions and a general anti-haemorrhagic.

Geranium maculatum Q.—To check instantly any kind of bleeding in alternation with *Ferrum phos.*

35. Hysteria

Occasional fainting and semi-unconciousness.

Camphor Q—Let the patient smell it to arouse from swoon.

Passiflora incarnata Q—To induce sleep.

Moschus Q—A general remedy.

Hydrocyanic acid Q—With convulsions and long gasping.

36. Hiccough

Ginseng Q, 1x—It is the specific remedy.

37. Heart Affections

Crataegus oxy Q—It is the specific remedy for all kinds of cardiac affections.

Cactus grand Q, 1x—Rheumatic heart with sense of constriction, as if screwed with iron hand, affection of left upper extermity.

Coccus cacti Q, 1x—Perverted action of the heart, stinging pains in the heart with haemorrhage of clotted blood from the heart.

Makaradhwaj Q, 1x—General tonic of heart, weak pulse.

Aconite nap Q—Weakness of heart with regular beat and imperceptible pulse, coldness of body, face cyanotic and like a corpse etc.

38. High Blood Pressure

Ranwolfia serpentina Q, 1x—A Specific remedy.

Nux vom 1x—In dyspeptics.

39. Insomnia

Loss of sleep.

Passiflora incarnata Q—60 drops is an ounce of hot water at 8 P.M. and if needed repeat at 9 P.M.

40. Insanity

Madness.

Ranwolfia serpantina Q, 1x—A specific remedy.

Passiflora—To induce sleep.

41. Impotency

Loss of power of sexual intercourse.

Avena sativa Q, Damiana Q and Ashwagandha Q—One dose each in 5 drop doses cures impotency, spermatorrhoea and nervous debility.

Camphor Q—It is a great stimulant but constant use causes importence. Similar is the action of *Cantharsis Q*.

42. Intermittent Fever

For exhaustive study read medicines in chapter 2 which have been written in chapter on Therapeutic Hints.

43. Jaundice

Paleness of urine, conjunctiva, constipation and biliousness.

Carduus marianus Q—A specific remedy.

Beberis vulgaris Q—If associated with kidney troubles originating in left kidney.

44. Kalaazar

Intermittent fever, blue distended veins, black tongue and

face, double rise of temperature, enlarged spleen and liver, tongue clean etc.

Kalmegh Q, 1x—It is a specific remedy.

Asai Q, 1x—In the last stage of Kalaazar with haematuria, bloody stool and affections of brain and heart are prominent.

Carduus Q—If liver complaints are prominent.

Ceanothus Q—To reduce the size of enlarged spleen.

45. Leprosy

It is characterised by red blotches, gangrene, numbness, tingling, deformities etc.

Jenocordia adorata Q, 1x—Specially useful in leprosy in the beginning stage.

Calopropis Q, 1x—Specially used in gangrenous stage.

Hydrocotyle asiatica Q, 1x—Red spots, circular spots with scaly edges.

Hygrophilla spinosa Q, 1x—Deep ulcers of leprosy.

Anacardium Q, 1x—Dr. Mahendra Lal Sirkar is reported to have cured a case of leprosy with *Anacardium*.

46. Labour Pain

Caulophyllum Q, 1x—Ensures painless delivery if given twice since seventh month. If given during labour it ensures safe delivery.

Passiflora incarnata Q—To reduce intolerable pain.

47. Leucorrhoea

Discharge of white yellow or reddish discharge from mucou membranes of uterus with backache and weakness.

Abroma augusta Q—Specially attended with dysmenorrhoea. Constipation, raveneous hunger, profuse and frequent micturition, intense thirst, etc.

Aletris ferinosa Q, 1x—Attended with weakness of uterus and general debility.

Ova tosta 1x—A well nigh specific attended with constant backache.

Asoka Q, 1x—With menstrual disorders.

Viburnum OP and Prun Q, 1x—Specially in those who are habituated to abortion or dysmenorrhoea.

48. Menstrual Disorders

Asoka Q—Is a specific remedy.

Senecio Q, 1x—Should be alternated with *Asoka Q*.

49. Mental Weakness

Weakness of memory attended with nervous debility and spermatorrhoea are radically cured by *Aswagandha Q*, and *Avena sativa Q*, 2 doses each in 5 drop doses. Abstain from coition till radical cure is gained.

50. Neuralgia

Pain in the course of nerves. Study *Pass avena, Passiflora incarnata* and *Passiflora* compound in second Chapter.

51. Nocturnal Emissions

Emission of semen at night in dream or without dream.

Ficcus indica Q, 1x—Spermatorrhoea due to excessive waste of semen.

Thymol Q, 1x—Attended with voluptuous fancies, frequent priapisms, prostatic discharge during micturitions.

Bellis perenis—If attended with vertigo.

52. Nervous Debility

Read *Aswagandha*, *Avena*, *Damiana* and *Alfalfa* in chapter II.

Origanum Q, 1x—If attended with excessive sexual excitement.

Mica Q, 1x—If due to excessive loss of blood and vital fluids.

Fluid cerefolius Q, 1x—Specially in old people with prostatic abnormality.

Salix nigra Q, 1x—If due to spermatorrhoea.

53. Night Blindness

Physostigma Q, 1x—Specific remedy. Also give *cod liver oil*.

54. Obesity (Fatness ; Corpulency).

Fucus vesiculosis Q, 1x—If attended with indigestion, flatulence.

Phytoline Q—Attended with difficulty in walking, sitting, palpitation, dyspnoea on the least exertion, nausea, eructations. A great fat reducer.

Esculentine Q—Another great fat reducer. May be alternated with *phytoline*.

55. Pthisis

It is characterised by pulmonary haemorrhage, excessive expectoration with pain, cavities in lungs, night sweats, teasing cough, fever in the evening, great emaciation and debility etc.

PTHISIS

Abrotanum Q, 1x – Pulmonary affections, rapid and great emaciation though eating well and ravenous hunger, emaciation ascending from feet upward, chilly, burning in stomach with indigestion and lack of assimilation.

Acalypha indica Q, 1x — Haemorrhage of bright red blood in the morning with that of dark and clotted blood in the afternoon, teasing incessant cough at night.

Jaborandi Q, 1x — It is very useful in profuse debilitating sweat at night in pthisis.

Nux Juglans Q, 1x — Cough, aphonia, heaviness in chest, distension and hardness of abdomen, diarrhoea, indigestion, glandular swelling with pus in axilla and its vicinity.

Natrum ars Q, 1x — Where symptoms of *Natrum mur* and *Arsenic* have combined.

Ficcus religiosa Q, 1x — Haemorrhage of bright red blood from lungs.

Blumia odorata Q, 1x — Of great service in pthisis with dry, barking, sawing cough, wheezing respiration, aphonia, hoarseness having history of haemorrhagic diathesis.

Hamamelis Q, 1x — Pulmonary haemorrhage of dark blood.

Cyndon Dactylon Q, 1x — In prominently haemorrhagic cases.

Justicia rubrum Q, 1x — Profuse haemorrhage from lungs with violent cough.

Occimum sanctum Q, 1x — First stage of consumptions with slight fever, distressing dry cough, expectoration of phlegm streaked with blood.

Eupatorium ayapan Q, 1x—Bleeding from lungs with cough in consumption.

56. Puerperal Fever

Chilliness, fever and other troubles in parturient mothers due to suppression of lochia producing a septic condition.

Asoka Q—To regulate the discharge of lochia.

Echinacea Q—Specific for puerperal fever.

57. Paralysis

Inability to use voluntary nerves with or without pain etc.

Nux vom Q, 1x—In the beginning of paralytic condition threatening tetanus.

Strychnia phos Q, 1x—If used in the very commencement it arrests the development of paralysis and cures it if used constantly for a considerably longer period.

58. Pits of Pox

Serracenia Q, 1x—It is a specific remedy to fill up the pits and scars caused by smallpox.

Variolinum—In high potency is another specific.

59. Palpitation of Heart

Avena sativa Q—If due to seminal losses and nervous breakdown.

Crataegus oxy Q—Specific remedy.

Asparagus ripens Q, 1x—See "Heart Affections".

60. Rheumatism and Gout

Pain, swelling and immobility of joints.

Hymosa Q. In acute febrile stage.

SNAKE BITE

Belladona Q, 1x — In stiffness and acute affections when the pains come and go like electric shockss, worse on touch and movement.

Viscum album Q — Rheumatism of joints of gonorrhoeal origin specially in women.

Passiflora incarnata Q — To reduce pain and induce sleep.

61. Snake Bite

Read *Leucus Aspera Echinacea* and *Eupatorium Ayapam* in chapter II.

62. Septicaemia

Blood poisoning.

Fluid calendula 1x — In all conditions it is a specific remedy.

Echinacea Q, 1x — Another best anti-septic.

Hemidesmus indica — A great blood purifier.

63. Supression of Urine.

Camphor Q — Suppression of urine and all discharges, dry skin, cold skin, aversion to covering, internal heat, faintness and imperceptible pulse.

Coleus Aromatics — Specific remedy.

64. Spermatorrhoea

Seminal loss, nocturnal emissions and consequent debility.

Avena sativa Q — One of the best medicines for mental, nervous, physical and seminal weakness.

Damiana Q — Similar as *Avena* and may be used alternatly.

Aswagandha Q — When mental weakness is prominent.

Ficcus Indica Q – When nocturnal emission is prominent.

Makaradhwaj Q—If associated with cardiac weakness.

Neuphar leuteum Q—Nocturnal emissions, impotence, early ejaculation and all affections dependent on them.

Saw palmeto Q—When enlargement of prostate is associated with spermatorrhoea.

Bellis parenis Q—Spermatorrhoea associated with vertigo.

Salix nigra Q—When impotence is prominent in spermatorrhoea.

65. Suppression of Milk

Ricinus Q— Internally and massage of it in the mamma is the best measure to induce secretion and increase of milk.

66. Senselessness

Fainting, unconsciousness sudden.

Amyl nitricum Q—Due to intense pain.

Camphor Q—Sudden fainting and unconsciousness with collapse etc.

Moschus Q—In unconsciousness of hysteria.

67. Skin Diseases

Calotropis gigentia Q, *1x*—Specially suitable for skin diseases, gangrenous ulcers with syphilitic poison.

Echinacea Q, *1x*—It is a specific remedy in all kinds of skin diseases in all stages due to accumulation of all kinds of miasmatic poisons. It is the best purifier of blood.

Spongia Q—It is regarded as a patent medicine for all kinds of skin diseases.

SPASMS

Cornus alternifolia Q—Specially for chilblains and broken skin.

68. Spasms

Painful contraction in the nerves.

Comphor Q—Spasms with dryness, internal heat and external coldness threatening collapse.

Passiflora incarnata or compound is specific remedy to relieve all kinds of spasms.

69. Syphilis

Ulcers of various kinds on genital organs, coppery red spots on skin in the primary stage and ulcer on tissues and bones of body in the later stage are main symptoms of syphilis.

Echinacea Q—In all kinds and stages of syphilis

Calotropis Q, 1x—In syphilis of advanced stage, resulting in leprosy of gangrenous type.

Cyndon dactylon Q, 1x—Specially in secondary syphilis with haemorrhagic diathesis and urinary troubles.

Cascara amarga Q—Prominent remedy in syphilis and may be alternated with *Echinacea*.

Hemidesmus indica Q—Very useful in syphilitic and other menifestations due to abuse of mercury associated with indigestion and loss of appetite.

Kali iod 1x—Syphilis suppressed in hot and sensitive patients.

70. Tremour

Trembling of head and limbs.

Agaricus Q— Associated with chorea and uterine disorders.

Nux vomica Q—Specially in persons of sedentary habit.

Tarentula Q—In tremour and uneasiness of limbs with cardiac or urinary troubles.

71. Tetanus

Convulsions with rigidity and curvature of spine etc.

Hypericum Q—Specially when injury to sentient nerves has caused tetanus.

Nux vom Q—Just in the beginning.

Strychnia Q—Acts like a patent medicine if given in the ver onset.

Passiflora compound Q—Immediately relieves pain and tension.

72. Tumour

Abnormal growth in the size of a nut or an egg.

Fraxinus americana Q—Useful for uterine tumours, fibrousy growths and distressing backache.

Hydrastis Q—In putrid tumours, threatening cancer.

Condurango Q—Tumours of cancerous dyscrasia.

Thuja Q—In sycotic subjects.

Chimaphilla Q—Chronic cystitis and violent pain and tumour of breasts.

73. Uterine Disorders

Aletris farinosa Q—General tonic and reformer of uterine troubles.

UTERINE DISORDERS

Hydrastis Q—Cancer, tumour of the uterus or leucorrhoeal discharges thick and yellow.

Asoka Q—It is the best regulator of menstrual troubles and all ailments dependent on them.

Viburnum Op and *Prunus* in all uterine ailments in women who are habituated to early abortion and dysmenorrhoea.

Note—For intensive study of medicines prescribed above, you must thoroughly study chapter II.

CHAPTER II

MATERIA MEDICA AND USE OF INTERNAL MOTHER TINCTURES

1. Abroma Augusta Q, 1x

Abroma augusta has gained high reputation in curing wonderfully diabetes mellitus and insipiduous. "Ravenous hunger, insatiable thirst, frequent and profuse micturition, obstinate constipation, indignant and forgetful disposition with rapidly growing extreme debility and pronounced emaciation" are the characteristic features of this wonderful Indian drug—*Ulat kamal*

It is an unique drug in the entire Materia Medica in affecting instant cure and relief in dysmenorrhoea. The patient creates panic by her shrieks and shrills due to intolerable pain, the blood is dark and clotted, sometimes yellowish with scanty or profuse menstrual flow. Chlorosis, hysteric spasms, irregular menses and leucorrhoea are the satellites revolving around dysmenorrhoea.

Direction : In diabetes adminster *Abroma Augusta* Q in 5 drop doses, 3 times a day and *Syzigium Jambolinum* (Jamun) *Q*, in 5 drops twice daily. In dysmenorrhoea and all complications associated with it give *Abroma augusta Q*, in 10 drop doses every hour or oftener according to the severity of the pain. During paroxysm *Passiflora incarnata Q*, should be given in 60 drop doses with an ounce of hot water at bed time to induce sleep.

After the cessation of menstrual period give *Abroma augusta 1x* in 2 drop doses, *Xanthoxyllum 1x* in 2 drop doses and *Asoka janosia Q*, in 5 drop-doses, each twice daily with an ounce of water. Continue this process till the next menstrual period. The treatment should continue utmost for 3 months according to method directed above.

To ensure radical cure give *Medorrhinum C.M.* 1 dose every month just after the menstrual period as most of the cases of dysmenorrhoea are dependent on sycotic, gonorrhoecal virus, contacted from husband.

2. Abroma Radix Q, 1x

It is prepared from the bark of *ulat kamal* whereas *Abroma augusta* is prepared from the leaves of the same Indian plant. *Abroma radix* is a great uterine tonic and is more efficacious than *Abroma augusta*. in all complaints especially dysmenorrhoea. It should be used in same way with all its complementary medicines.

3. Abrotanum 1x

I agree with Dr. Johns in affirming that this drug affects marvelous cure of consumption with peritonitis, emaciation and marasmus from feet upward with constant distention and acidity in the abdomen, face shrivelled, dry cold and pale with the characteristics that the patient loses flesh rapidly while living well with ravenous hunger like *Iodin, Natrum mur*. Give 1x in 2 drop doses 4 times a day or according to the severity of the case. This drug may be complemented with *Tuberculinum* 1M. once in a month.

4. Acalypha Indica Q, 1x

This drug has gained universal reputation in the domain of homoeopathy for its wonderful efficacy in affecting instant relief and radical cure in the haemorrhage from lungs in consumptives with the characteristics :

"Haemorrhage of bright red blood in the morning and that of dark clotted blood in the afternoon; and soreness and teasing incessant cough at night."

To be used in Q, in the beginning in 5 drop doses 4 times a day in an ounce of cool water and afterwards 1x in 2 drop doses 4 times a day.

Complementaries—*Blumia odorata, Ficcus religiosa, Hamamelis, Aconite nap, Phosphorus,* etc.

5. Aeglafolia—Bilwapatra Q, 1x

It is a very efficacious remedy in all kinds of local and general dropsy, anasarsca, or ascites with or without fever, diarrhoea or constipation, with full soft and regular pulse.

The mother tincture of this wonderful drug should be used in 5 drop doses two times a day and this should be alternated with *Borrhavia difussa Q* in 5 drop-doses twice daily in dropsies. Persons desirous to maintain celebacy with calmness of libido should use *Aeglefolia Q* in 2 drop doses twice daily with an ounce of cool water.

Aeglefolia 200, once in a week removes impotency, restores sexual strength and vitality.

6. Aegla Marmelos –Bilwa Fal Q, 1x

It is equally efficacious in all complaints amenable to *Aegla folia*. It is very efficacious in diarrhoea and dysentery, in acute and chronic stages in children, young men and the fragile old persons when *Merc-cor.*, etc. have failed.

Use from 5 to 20 drops a dose in cool water at intervals of 2 to 3 hours according to the severity of the case.

7. Aconite Radix 1x

It acts like a magic in "thin, watery stools, vomiting of green, black and bilious substance, violent tenesmus and pain in abdomen, retention of urine, coldness and blueness of the whole body, respiration very difficult and cold, vertigo, pulse feeble, imperceptible."

Use this remedy in 1x dilution in 1 drop-dose with cool water at intervals of every 15 minutes. In case of senselessness or inability to swallow the remedy, let the patient inhale the remedy purely droped in cotton and it will prove to be a great saviour. In chilliness, shivering and perspiration during tetanic convulsions give *Aconite radix 1x*, 1 drop with an ounce of cool water, every 15 minutes.

8. Aconite Nap Q, 1x

This wonderful drug has saved many lives from inevitable death in the stage of collapse with "coldness of body, face cyanotic and like a corpse, great agony, restlessness, fear of death, weakness of heart with regular beat but imperceptible pulse."

Give *Aconite* Q in 1 drop dose with cool water every 15 minutes.

In rheumatic fever when the temperature rises higher than 105°, give *Aconite* Q drop in cool water every 15 minutes and the temperature will sooner come down to normalcy.

Rubini's *Camphor* Q and *Cimicifuga* Q likewise act as a magic in getting the high temperature of rheumatic fever down in 2 to 5 drop doses, the former with sugar of milk and the latter in an ounce of cool water.

9. Acenasia Q

"Great languor, cold perspiration on the whole body fetid breath, ulcers in pharynx, diphtheria and haemorrhage of dark blood," call for its use in 5 to 10 drop doses every 2 nours.

It may be complemented with a dose of *Diphtherinum* 200 in malignant diphtheria.

10. Acid Hydro. 1x to 3x

In collapse stage when the death is threatening with the following symptoms :

"Sunken eyes and face, face cyanotic like a corpse, whole body like a corpse, cold and wet with cold sweat, blueness of nails and forepart of nails shrivelled, senselessness or groaning, moaning, water or medicine does not descend from throat, imperceptible pulse, very slow respiration, great difficulty in breathing, the patient has to gasp for a few seconds for taking breath as if this is the last attempt, half open eyes or staring look."

Give 1x, 2x or 3x in 2 drop doses plain on the tongue every 5 minutes.

11. Arsenic Alb, 3x

In suppression of urine in cholera, with great torpor, delirium, and restlessness give *Ars. alb. 3x* one drop every hour or oftener. A single dose of *Ars. alb. 3x trit.* will aggravate the suppressed malarial fever and cure the patient from all ailments due to suppression of ague with quiuine.

12. Anacardium 1x

In elephantiasis give *Anacardium 1x*, 1 drop thrice daily on failure of *Hydrocotyle Asiatica*. Complement this with the well selected remedy according to totality of the symptoms of the patient.

13. Aloes Q

It is efficacious in dysenteric stools with mucous and blood with prolapsus ani, loss of control over sphincter ani, and consequent passage of frequent involuntary stools, and anus wide.

2 drops with cool water 4 times a day.

14. Apocynum Q

General anasarca, chilly patient, intense thirst with frequent watery stools, vomiting, free micturition in ratio of the intake of water.

15. Agaricus Q

It is the most important remedy for chorea, twitching, tingling of muscles, tremor of head and electric like shocks in the spinal column. Give 5 drops in an ounce of cool water thrice daily.

16. Aletris Farinosa Q

This is a great uterine tonic. It is one of the most valuable remedies to cure uterine disorders. It is successfully used in the weakness of the uterus caused by frequent child bearing and over work.

In insufficient menstrual flow and leucorrhoea associated with debility and anaemia, it works miraculously. Give *Aletris farinosa* in 5 drop doses twice daily and alternate with *Asoka janosia* Q in 5 drop doses twice daily. This will bring tone to the uterus and remove all irregularity of menses and complaints dependent on it.

In leucorrhoea *Aletris* Q likewise should be alternated with *Ova testa 3x* in 3 grains doses twice daily, with a dose or two of *Viburnum opulus* Q.

In uterine displacement and prolapsus uteri this drug should be used twice daily in Q dilution in 5 drop doses and simultaneously *Viburnum opulus* should be administered. *Viburnum prunifolia* Q should be alternated with *Altris* Q in habitual abortion of women in the same manner.

In sterility and chlorosis its constant use renders uterus free from all defects and enables sterile women to give birth to alive children. If sterility be dependent on obesity, *Phytoline* Q in 10 drop doses should be used twice daily. In functional sterility it should be given twice daily alternated with *Corpus leuteum* 3x, 2 tabs a dose thrice daily.

Aletris farinosa Q is specially useful in gastic derrangement connected with uterine disorders or in pregnant women such as loss of appetite. distention of abdomen after the fat food, disgust for food, nausea and constipation as well as fainting fits with vertigo.

In these cases *Aletris Q*, 5 drops in cool water thrice daily is very beneficial and it should be alternated with *Carica papaya 1x*, 2 drops or 2 grains a dose twice daily after meals.

It has been successfully used in obstinate vomiting of pregnancy. *Aletris Q*, 5 drops twice daily in cool water alternated with *Symphcricarpus racemosa Q*, 5 drops twice daily act like magic in stopping and curing obstinate vomiting of pregnancy.

17. Amyl Nitric Q

In sudden senselessness and unconsciousness in epileptic convulsions, let the patient smell at *Amyl nitric Q* and it will bring him back to sense.

Similarly let the patient inhale *Amyl nitric Q* in unbearable, fatal pain and it will pacify him.

18. Arnithogallum Ambeletum Q, 1x

Give a single dose of this remedy *Q*, 2 drops with an ounce of cool water in gastric ulcer and it will act wonderfully. If necessary repeat the dose after a long interval.

19. Alfalfa Q

Alfalfa is a great tissue builder and greatly increases weight. It is highly efficacious in anaemia, chlorosis, marasmus, deficient development, pthisis and all conditions characterised by tissue waste. It is likewise successfully used in convalescence, after child birth and during lactation.

Dose—Half to one tea-spoonful in an ounce of water, milk or tea 3 times a day, less for children according to age.

In convalescence after serious acute diseases such as pneumonea, typhoid etc. *Psorinum 200*, single dose should be given along with *Alfalfa* to expedite the restoration of strength and vigour and prevent recurrence of the disease.

20. Avena Sativa Q

This remedy is pre-eminently nutrient to the nervous system. It is stimulant and great builder, and restorative to nervous power. It is a most wonderful remedy in all cases of nervous exhaustion, general debility. In such cases, *Avena sativa Q*, 5 drops in cool water thrice daily is very beneficial. In nervous palpitation of the heart it should be used twice daily in an ounce of cool water and should be alternated with *Crataegus oxy Q*, 5 drops in cool water twice daily.

In insomnia with despondency it should be given twice daily in 5 drop doses in cool water added with a dose of *Passiflora incarnata Q* 60 drops in an ounce of hot water at bed time.

It is very useful in weakness of memory and inability to fix his attention on any subject while thinking or reading with mental, nervous and physical debility due to excessive indulgence in onanism and masturbation. In such cases specially in students and mental workers of modern age, **mix** *Avena sativa, Aswagrandha* and *Damiana* all in *Q* dilution, each 2 drops in an ounce of cool water and use thrice daily for a month or more and abstain from sexual intercourse for at least 2 months and see the miracles of these drugs.

AVENA SAVITA

It is likewise efficacious beyond expectation in nervous exhaustion of women due to excessive indulgence in sexual intercourse with mental depression and physical prostration with amenorrhoea, violent pain in pelvic region, emission of phosphates and other white substances in the urine, pain in occiput etc.

In all such cases *Avena satvia* 3 drops in an ounce of cool water thrice daily should be used and alternated with *Asoka janosia Q* twice daily in 5 drop doses with an ounce of cool water.

Avena sativa is a specific for curing the *morphine* or *opium* eating. The patient should lessen the quanity of *opium* gradually. It should be given in hot water 15 drops four times a day and the patient will do without eating *opium* in a short span of time.

To eradicate and eliminate abnormalities of *opium* it is advisable to take a dose of *Plumbum 200*, single dose and this will cure the patient from any kind of ailment due to long and constant use of *opium*. *Avena sativa* will get rid him of the morphine habit and increase and add new vigour in his exhausted nervous system.

In the treatment of enlargement of the prostrate it forms avaluable auxiliary of saw palmetto. In the treatment of sexual debility, spermatorrhoea and nocturnal emissions it should be used as an alternative with *Salix nigra* or 3 drops of each should be mixed in an ounce of cool water and given thrice daily.

In the treatment of impotence mix 3 drops of *Avena sativa Q* with 3 drops of *Damiana Q* in an ounce of cool water and give thrice daily for a long time.

21. Asoka Janosia Q

Asoka janosia has gained universal reputation as a great saviour of women from all ailments peculiar to the fair sex. Why should any woman suffer so long this great saviour survives on the earth ?

It is a great uterine tonic with the greatest efficacy in all uterine and menstrual disorders. Its action is certain and surpasses all alike remedies. It can be used as a principal remedy or alternated with other remedies similar to it in usefulness. "Violent pain in pelvic region due to sudden suppression of menstrual flow with extention of this pain in the whole abdominal region, and violent pain in head and lumbar region. Commencement of menstrual flow is preceded by violent pain in pelvic cavity, flow thin, watery or yellowish or discharge of black fetid blood, most inveterate cases of chronic leucorrhoea with sterility. Intense pain in lower abdomen, very fetid, long lasting black lochia.

Thirst, weakness; vertigo, diarrhoea etc. due to uterine disorders, great debility and pronounced emaciation, palpitation of heart, intense intolerable pain and burning during micturition, anaemia ; chlorosis, in lean and thin hysteric woman."

Principally in these ailments *Asoka Q* 5 drop doses thrice daily should be used and it must be used as an intercurrent remedy and complementary to *Abroma augusta, Xanthoxyllum, Aletris ferinosa, Viburnum opulus, Viburnum prunifolia, Ova testa, Pulsatilla, Sepia, Cimicifuga, Caulophyllum* etc. with grand success.

22. Arjun—Terminalia Arjuna Q

It is a great heart tonic.

"Feeling as if something has prevented the movement of heart and it would stop beating at any moment ; palpitation of heart so violent that the patient faints and gives up hope of life. He is obliged to lie on the left side pressing hard in hope of relief.

Feeling as if too much blood has accumulated in the heart and expects relief if vomiting of blood takes place. Piercing in the heart with violent palpitation before coughing. Pulse very irregular, sometimes very quick and sometimes very feeble and slow."

In these characteristic symptoms *Arjun* is the greatest saviour It should be used in Q dilution in 5 drop doses thrice daily and alternated with *Crataegus oxy* Q twice daily in 5 drop doses, both with an ounce of cool water.

23. Atista Indica Q

Atista Indica is beneficial in all kinds of worms and ailments dependent on them. Pain around navel due to round worms (*Cina, Santonine*), itching inside the nose and tendency to boring finger in the nostrils (*Cina*).

Convulsions and fever due to worms. Itching in anus due to small thread worms (*Tellureum*). It is alone efficient to expel and kill all kinds of worms and should be given in Q dilution in 2 to 5 drop doses in an ounce of cool water.

Atista Indica is also very beneficial in intermittent fever recurring every 3rd day or 4th day with chilliness, thirst in the stage of heat, white coating on tongue, burning in liver and spleen in the evening. In intermittent fever *Atista*, 2 drops in an ounce of cool water should be given 4 times a day.

It is very beneficial in all sorts of diarrhoea and dysentery.

24. Atista Radix 1x

In all complaints it is equally beneficial like *Atista Indica*, but in dysentery with bloody stools, convulsions in children, fever, diarrhoea, pain in abdomen and worms *Atista radix 1x*, is more efficacious.

It should be used in 1 drop doses 4 times a day.

25. Asai

Marvellous results are obtained by this drug in the last stage of Kalaazar when haematuria and bloody stools are prominent and when the heart and brain effections exhibit their supremacy in last stage of Kalaazar.

Asai 1x or *3x* should be used in one drop doses 4 times a day. It may be complemented with *Hamamelis* Q 5 drops twice daily in haemorrhage from bladder and intestines. After a bit relief this drug should be alternated with *Kalmegh* Q 5 drops twice daily. If necessary *Ceanothus* Q 5 drops twice daily should be also given.

26. Azadirecta Indica, 1x

In chronic malarial fever, the liver and spleen are enlarged and indurated, paroxysm of fever in the evening with bilious complaints with cough and burning in the eyes specially when the ague is suppressed with overdose of quinine.

Chill : Rise of temperature with slight chill in the afternoon.

Heat : Burning in eyes, face, palms and soles, relief in open cool air.

Sweat : Slight sweat on upper parts, only. Scanty sweat or absence of it. It is very beneficial in fever with burning, thirstlessness, gonorrhoea and spermatorrhoea.

It is also useful in skin diseases and leprosy. Give this drug in 1x or 3x dilutions, 4 times a day in one drop doses.

27. Andersonia Rohitak Q 1x

This remedy has proved its efficacy in acute as well as chronic malaria.

Chill : Paroxysm of chill at about 4 P.M.

Heat : Vertigo before chill. Intense burning and flashes of heat in palms, soles, face, eyes, dryness of mouth, intense thirst for cool water and violent nausea after drinking.

Sweat : Absence of perspiration.

Prodormal Stage : Bitter taste in the mouth, pain in enlarged spleen and liver, pulse full and bounding.

Constipation with dry and hard stools. Give *Andersonia rohitak Q* in 5 drop doses thrice daily in the beginning and then in 1x dilution in 1 drop doses thrice daily.

28. Aswagandha Q

Aswagandha is a great mental tonic. It acts like a magic in slowly advancing mental inertia, imbecility, with loss of comprehension and expression. Likewise it is beneficial in the loss of memory. In short *Aswagandha Q* is highly efficacious in total or partial destruction of intellect, where the power of thinking, memory and expression is paralysed.

For a student who cannot fix his attention on any subject nor can memorise his lessons, nor express what he has read, *Aswagandha* is a great friend.

In co-ordination of muscular power with spermatorrhoea, weakness of nerves and muscles due to gout, syphilis and gonorrhoea call for the constant use of *Aswagandha* for a long time. It acts like a magic in impotence and all kinds of seminal deficiencies. General weakness, sterility, leucorrhoea, menstrual disorder, haemorrhage in women, all are amenable to this drug.

Use in 5 drop doses thrice daily in alternation with other indicated remedies.

29. Alstonia Scholaris Q 1x

It is a great remedy for malaria fever—and more efficacious than *quinine*. It checks all kinds of intermittent fever more quickly than *quinine*. *Quinine* always suppresses malaria and is solely responsible for all untoward results due to the suppression of malaria. *Alstonia* never suppresses ague rather cures it permanently with no after-effects.

Alstonia is a great tonic for weakness—and rundown constitution due to suffering malaria or other fevers for a long time. It is an unique remedy in digestive disorders, diarrhoea and dysentery concomitant with malarial fever. Give *Alstonia Q* in 5 drop doses thrice daily in the beginning and 1x in one drop doses thrice daily.

30. Asparagus Officinalis 1x

It is of great service in the following complaints :

Affections of the heart : Violent palpitation of heart, pain in the heart, aggravation on walking. Dysponea due to hydrothorax. Difficult deglutition in hydrophobia. "Passage of stones in urine, severe toothache". Thrice daily in one drop doses.

31. Absinthium Q 1x

It is of great service in epileptiform seizures preceded by nervous tremors. Sudden and nervous giddiness, delirium with hallucinations and loss of consciousness. Nervous excitement and sleeplessness. It is likewise very efficacious in cerebral irritation, hysteria and infantile spasms, chorea, tremor, nervousness, excitement and sleeplessness in children.

Give *Absinthium Q*, 2 to 4 drops or *1x* 1 drop during paroxysm every 10 to 15 minutes ; otherwise 4 times a day.

32. Adonis Vernalis Q

It is one of the most valuable heart medicine in all kinds of heart affections preceded by rheumatism or influenza or Bright's disease when the functional power of heart and the urinary organs have diminished. It is a most valuable remedy in cardiac dropsy, hydrothorax, ascites, anasarca, low vitality with weak heart and slow, weak pulse. Give 5 to 10 drops of the tincture 4 times a day.

33. Agave Americana Q

It is a very effective remedy in gonorrhoea with painful erection like *Cantharis*, with strangury. It is indicated in pain in stomach with poor appetite and constipation. It is also useful in scurvy, countenance pale, gums swollen and bleeding with legs covered with dark purple blotches, swollen, painful and hard. Give 5 drops of tincture thrice daily.

34. Alunus Q

It is useful in indigestion from impartial secretion of gastric juice. It stimulates nutrition and thus acts favourably in strumous disorders and cures enlarged glands. It is of equal value in leucorrhoea, with erosions of cervix, bleeding easily, and it is beneficial in amenorrhoea with burning pain from back to pubis. Give 5 drops of tincture thrice daily.

35. Ambrosia Q

It is a valuable remedy in the folllowings :—Hay fever, lachrimation and intolerable itching of the eyelids, whooping cough with wheezing respiration. Respiratory tracts in its entire length stopped up, stuffed feeling in nose and head. Nose bleed. Irritation of trachea and bronchial tubes, with asthmatic attacks. Give 10 drops of tincture in an ounce of water during and after attacks of epistaxis.

In other cases 5 drops of tincture 4 times a day.

36. Amygdatus Persica Q

A most valuable remedy in vomiting of various kinds, constant nausea and vomiting, morning sickness of pregnancy.

It is very efficacious in gastric irritation of children, food of any kind is not tolerated. Loss of smell and taste. Gastric and intestinal irritation when the tongue is elongated and pointed tip and edges red.

Give 2 drops of tincture every 2 hours or thrice daily.

37. Apocynum Androsacimicfolium Q

The rheumatic symptoms of this remedy promise most curative results. Its pain are of wandering nature with much stiffness and drawing. Trembling and prostration. Pain in all joints. Pain in toes and soles.

Swelling of hands and feet. Tingling pain in toe. Cramps in soles. Violent heat in soles.

Give 5 drops of tincture in an ounce of water 4 times a day.

38. Apomorphia 1x

Its hypodermic injection 1 drop of 1x, with 15 drops of sterile water acts as a safe and sure hypnotic. Acts well in delirium and insomnia. Sleep comes on in half an hour. Do not repeat the injection.

39. Agnilegia 1x

A good remedy in hysteria globus and clavus hystericus. Sleeplessness. Nervous trembling of body, sensitive to noise and light.

Dysmenorrhoea of young girls. Menses scanty, with dull, painful nightly increasing pressure in the right lumbar region.

Give 5 drops of tincture thrice daily.

40. Aralia Racemosa Q

One of the best remedies for asthmatic conditions with cough aggravated on laying down. Dry cough coming on after first sleep about middle of night. Asthma on lying down with spasmodic cough; worse after first sleep with tickling in throat.

Hay-fever; frequent sneezing. Rawness and burning behind sternum. The least current of air causes sneezing with copious watery excoriating nasal discharge, of salty acrid taste.

Likewise it is curative in suppression of menses, suppression of lochia with tympanitis, leucorrhoea foul smelling, acrid, with pressing down pain.

Give *Aralia race.* Q 5 drops 4 times a day.

41. Arania Diadema Q

It is a very useful remedy in intermittent fever with swollen spleen with following characteristics :—

All symptoms of *Arania* are characterised by periodicity and coldness and great susceptibility to dampness. It is the remedy for the constitution with the favourable to malarial poisoning when every damp day or place favours chilliness. Patient feels cold to the very bone. Hydrogenoid constitution *i.e.*, abnormal sensitiveness to damp and cold, inability to live near fresh water, lakes, rivers etc. or in damp, marshy chilly places (*Natr. Sul, Thuja*) coldness not relieved by any thing.

Besides these it is of great service in sensation as if hands are twice their normal size after walking. Feeling as if parts were enlarged and heavier. Coldness with pain in long hours and feeling of stone in abdomen at the same hour daily. Chilly day and night, always worse during rain. Give five drops of tincture thrice daily.

42. Arbutus Andrachev Q

It is a valuable remedy for eczema associated with gouty and rheumatic symptoms, arthritis specially larger joints, lumbago. Symptoms shift from skin to joints. Give 5 drops of tincture thrice daily.

43. Arsenic Bromatum Q

It has proved a great anti-psoric and anti-syphilitic remedy. Herpetic eruptions, syphilitic excresoences, glandular tumours and induration carcinoma, locomotor ataxia and obstinate intermittents and diabetes all are cured by this drug. Tincture 3 drops thrice daily.

44. Asclepias Syriaca Q

It principally acts on nervous system and burning organs. A great remedy for dropsy, hepatic, renal and cardiac and post-scarlatinal affections. A great diaphoretic and augments the urinary secretion. Acute reheumatic inflammation of the large joints. Tincture 5 drops thrice daily.

45. Aspidosperma 1x

Dr. Hale regards it as the digitalis of the lungs. It removes temporary obstruction to the oxidation of the blood by stimulating respiratory centres increasing oxidation and excretion of carbonic acid. Pulmonary, stenosis thrombosis of pulmonary artery. Uraemic dyspnoea. An effective remedy in many cases of asthma. It stimulates the respiration centres and incrcases the oxygen in the blood.

Cardiac asthma. Want of breath during exertion is the guiding symptom. Give tincture 5 drops every hour or 1x, trit, one grain every hour.

46. Aurum Mur. Natronatum 3

This remedy has most pronounced effect on the female organs and Burnett is of opinion that it has more power over uterine tumours than any other remedy. It is useful in indurated cervix, chronic metritis, prolapsus. Uterus fills up whole pelvis. Sub-involution, ossified uterus. Ovarix indurated.

Ovarian dropsy, ulceration of cervix uteri and vaginae. It is also useful in psoriasis syphilieait. Swelling of testicles. Syphilitic ataxia. 1 grain to be given thrice daily.

47. Asarum Europium 3x

It is of great service in pregnancy of early months in vomiting of whatever is taken in nervous women who are oversensitive to even the sound produced by fiction of paper or cloth. Give 3x, 2 drops 4 times a day.

48. Amalki Q

Mix the juice of *Amla* part 1 in 1 part of alcohol and the mother tincture is prepared. It is of great service in nocturnal emissions spermatorrhoea and cough. It also turns the grey hair to complete blackness. Give Q 3 drops thrice daily.

49. Aqua-Ptychosis Q

It is a very valuable remedy in digestive disorders, indigestion, dyspepsia, flatulence, diarrhoea and heart-burn. Give Q 5 drops, 4 times a day.

50. Achyranthus Asperalin Q 1x

Frequent, painless, watery profuse involuntery stools with vomiting, prostration, intense thirst, retention of urine and feeble pulse are the characteristic of this drug. Burning in stomach, sour eructations, occasional nausea and vomiting of water phlegm with intense thirst, drinks often but little at a time and the water is ejected as soon as it is taken with daily in an ounce of cool water complemented with *Aswagandha* twice daily in 5 drop doses.

In paralytic affections, convulsions with insomnia dependent on masturbation it is the remedy. In bubo and cancer of the breasts it surpasses *Phytolacca* and aids as an complementary to it.

In whitlows after blow, the pain ascends upward from the site of blow. In convulsions of children with starting, it is like *Belladonna* with absence of red eyes and face dilated pupils and throbbing of the carotides. Give *Bufo Q* 5 drops thrice or 4 times daily.

62. Berberis Vulgaris Q

It is serviceable in hepatic and renal disorders with pain in liver and abdomen with gravel in the kindney. In intolerable pain of renal colic it gives instant relief after failure of *Calcarea carb*. In hepatic congestion with pain in urethra, thigh, lumbar region and groins, in jaundice due to renal calculi and severe pain during the passage of calculi, it acts like a magic and cures the patient permanently in a very short period of time. In all ailments give *Berberis Q* 5 drops every hour or oftener according to the severity of the case in mild form give thrice daily.

63. Bellis Perennis Q

It acts like a magic in nocturnal emissions, spermatorrhoea, discharge of prostratic fluid in the urine, vertigo consequent on masturbation. Give *Bellis* Q 5 drops twice daily and *Thuja Q* 5 drops twice daily each in an ounce of cool water.

64. Baptisia Q, 1x

In malarial fever due to inhaling of fetid odour of faeces, poisonous air of ditches with rapid prostration; temperature above 105°-107° violent headache; furious delirium; and a feeling as if the limbs were apart from him and an attempt to gather the scattered limbs, it acts like a magic. It is likewise efficacious in putrid fever in typhoil state with temperature 103°-105°, watery, very offensive black stools; foul smell in breath and body, tongue dry and dirty. In typhoid state in any disease specially in bloody and mucus dysentry with fetid odour in the faeces *Baptisia Q* is the remedy. Give *Baptisia Q* 3 drops every 2 hours or oftener.

65. Belladonna Q

In opium poisoning, when the patient is unconscious and drifting towards death, give purgative and evacuate poisons through vomiting and stools. After that give *Belladonna Q* 10 drops in an ounce of hot water every half an hour and oftener. Then give *Vinegar* in hot water. Avoid sleep. In stiff-neck when the pains come and go like electric shocks with intermittency *Belladonna 1x* 2 drops every 3 hours is well nigh specific.

66. Caladium Seguinum Q

Caladium is a powerful remedy in asthma alternating with itching, burning rash, asthma with relief when the mucus is raised. It is very efficacious in spermatorrhoea, nocturnal emissions, and importence. It diminishes the craving for tobacco. Intolerable itching in genital organs is easily amenable to

CAMPHOR

Caladium. Give 2 to 5 drops of the tincture in an ounce of boiled water after meals and at bed time.

67. Camphor Q

Adapted to sudden diseases. It acts as a stimulant. It is principally used in coldness of body with profuse sweats collapse and feeble pulse. Rapid sinking of strength; spasms, violent convulsions, face pale, congestive chills, cholera infantum with sudden vomiting and diarrhoea, cholera asiatica with collapse, sun stroke etc. In extreme coldness of body it can be rubbed on skin. In convulsions of children let it smell at *Camphor*. *Camphor* give in 5 drop doses.

It is a sexual excitent and porlongs retentive power during coition. If taken regularly it cures impotence. Give 5 drops in sugar of milk every minute to an hour according to the nature of the case. Give a dose of *Camphor Q* 5 drops with sugar in acute coryza. Use *Camphor* with full faith in collapse stage of smallpox, in rheumatic fever when the temperature exceeds 105°, in feeble and irregular pulse, in any disease, in acute endocarditis, in "spasmodic stricture of urethra, in sudden retention of urine with burning and distress." *Camphor* acts like a magic in paroxysm of hysteria; let the patient smell at *Camphor*.

68. Carduus Marianus Q

Carduus acts principally on the liver. It is beneficial in hepatic congestion due to cold or alcoholic drinks. When the action of the liver is sluggish, the secretion of bile is insufficient and causes jaundice, the bowels constipated, motions clay coloured and the tongue foul with a feeling of langour and general debility. It works like a magic in cirrhosis of the liver due to alcoholic habits and cures all the complaints dependent on it viz. gastric derangements, vomiting of blood, jaundice scanty urination, dropsy etc. It removes all ailments such as torpidity and induration of liver, gall stone colic, inflammation of the hepatic region. In any disease if constipation is prominent, give *Carduus* 1 in one drop doses intercurrently with the indicated remedy. It will give tone to the liver, remove constipation and aid in rapid cure of the case.

Stools of *Carduus* are black, hard like balls in knots, like clay and without colour of the bile.

Dr. Ambers advocates for the use of *Chelidonium Q* and Dr. Birjosky lays stress on the use of *Carduus Q* in gall-stone colic and affirms that constant use of *Carduus* prevents recurrence of gall-stone colic and formation of bile-stones and thereby cures gall-stone colic permanently as it is possessed of all virtues to crrect the disorders of the liver.

Jaundice dependent on gall-stones is also amenable to *Carduus*.

Carduus exerts a curative action also on the spleen, in conditions similar to those of the liver. The diseases of the two organs are concurrent. In such cases *Carduus* should be alternated with *Ceanothus Americanus Q*.

Chronic congestion and cirrhosis of liver give rise to piles. In these conditions *Carduus* should be administered.

Vericose veins, also vericose ulcers, whether complicated

with the diseases of the liver and spleen or is not cured by *Carduus*.

Dr. Windelband of Berlin records the cure of 145 cases out of 190 vericose veins with this remedy. *Hamamelis*, *Sulphur* and *Fluoric acid* should be used intercurrently in vericose veins.

Give *Carduus Q*, 5 drops thrice daily. In emergency case give every hour or oftener.

69. Cascara Amarga Q

This remedy has a specific action on syphilis in all its stages and development. It cures the disease by purifying the blood.

Give *Cascara Q* 5 drops twice daily and *Echinacea Q* 5 drops each twice daily with an ounce of cool water.

70. Ceanothus Americanus Q

In the enlargement of spleen and liver *Ceanothus* is specific and has gained universal reputation. It likewise cures enlargement of spleen and liver due to other causes. The more enormously large is the spleen, the more *Ceanothus* is beneficial. It surpasses all other remedies in acute and chronic splenitis, and a deep seated pain in the left hypochondrium.

Give *Ceanothus Q* 2 to 5 drops three times a day and alternate it with *Carduus Q* in the same way.

If enlargement of spleen is due to Kala-azar alternate it with *Kalmegh Q* 2 to 5 drops twice daily.

In splenitis give *Ceanothus 1* one drop thrice daily. Also paint one part of Q with 9 parts of olive oil on the region of spleen.

71. Convallaria Majalis Q

Convallaria corrects irregularities of the heart due to vulvular diseases especially mitral pericardial adhesions etc. rather than tissue degeneration. It calms the heart, renders its movements rhythmical and slows the pulse. It cures dropsy caused by the sluggish action of the heart. It cures palpitation, dyspnoea, diminished secretion of urine, oedema of the feet etc., due to inability of the circulatory system. Give *Convallaria* Q 5 drops in an ounce of cool water thrice daily and *Crataegus oxy* Q 5 drops twice daily.

72. Crataegus Oxyacantha Q

It is the most important heart tonic. It is the safest remedy in all kinds of heart affections. It is the best remedy for heart failure due to organic vulvular diseases or anaemia of tissue degeneration. It slows and strengthens the pulse, makes breathing free and increases the secretion of urine and relieves dropsy.

It is the most effecacious remedy in angina pectoris, palpitation of heart and breathing due to least exertion or excitement. Intolerable pain of angina pectoris extends to left arm. It is likewise curative in the rheumatism of the heart but if this be the result of suppression of the rheumatism alternate with the indicated remedy. It acts like a magic in organic as well as functional derangement of the heart. Englargement and dilation of heart with pulse quick, feeble, irregular and intermittent are ameneble to it. Give *Crataegus* 10 to 15 drops in an ounce of warm water every 10 to 15 minutes in emergency cases, otherwise daily in the same manner.

73. Cactus Grandifolius Q

It has a direct action on heart, sensation as if the heart is squeezed with an iron hand. The same feeling is present in the throat, chest, rectum, bladder, uterus, and vagina. With this feeling, it acts like a magic, in great prostration, debility, total loss of strength, in neuralgic pains, constant redness and dejection. Give Q 5 drops thrice daily.

74. Coccus Cacti Q

It is a specific remedy in whooping cough and consequent convulsions. Sensation as if a hair or a thread is lying in the throat with titilation followed by paroxysms of suffocative cough, especially after rising from sleep, then expectoration of thick, sticky, phlegm. Perverted condition of the heart, stinging pains in heart with haemorrhage of clotted blood from the heart. In these affections give *Coccus Q* 5 drops thrice daily complemented with *Crataegus Q* 10 drops twice daily.

75. Chaparo Amargosa Q

It acts like a magic in the most chronic diarrhoea when all indicated remedies fail. Give Q in 2 to 4 drop doses 3 to 4 times a day.

76. Cenic Cio Q

It is beneficial in all kinds of menstrual disorders,

Give *Cenicio Q* 5 drops thrice daily and *Asoka Q* 5 drops twice daily.

77. Castor Oil Q

In dysentery of children it acts like a magic. Give *Castor oil* pure in one drop dose 3 times a day and *Aegle marmelos* Q 20 drops twice daily. In obstinate constipation and other ailments dependent on it give *Caster oil* pure 5 drops in an ounce of cool water at bed time.

The author has cured a case of gastric ulcer by constant use of this drug in 5 drop doses associated with constipation.

78. Chirata Q

It is very efficacious remedy in curing malarial fever and more efficacious when associated with scabies and other eruptions.

Violent shaking chill in the morning lasting for a long time, followed by heat lasting for 3 to 4 hours with thirst, nausea and vomiting. From 2 to 4 P.M. absence of chill and nominal heat with flashes of heat from eyes.

Give 5 drops or 1x, 2 drops thrice daily.

79. Coffea Mocha Q

It is a specific remedy for cholera. Give 10 drops in an ounce of water every 10 minutes and 3 doses are more than sufficient.

80. Cubeba Q

It gives instant relief and cures permanently the affections of gonorrhoea in the first inflammatory stage with dischage of thick yellow pus and burning in urethra during micturition. Give it 5 drops thrice daily and *Xasicaria com* 5 drops twice daily in an ounce of cool water.

81. Cannabis Sativa Q

In acute stage of gonorrhoea, it is very efficacious in the **inflammation of the bladder, thin** scanty pus, intense burning

CANNABIS

and pain and the patient walks with legs apart. Give *Cannabis Q* 5 drops thrice daily. *Thuja* 30 one dose a day and *Natrum sulph 6x* twice daily. In asthma when the patient can breath easily only in the standing position alternate it with *Blata orientalis Q*, 5 drops twice daily each.

82. Cannabis Indica Q

Dr. Cowperthwaite suggests to give *Cannabis indica Q* 3 drops thrice daily in violent pain of hemicrania of any side.

83. Croton Tig Q

In obstinate constipation *Croton tig* is a marvellous remedy. Prepare *Croton tig Q* by mixing 1 part of *croton oil* with 1 part of *Alcohal*. Give one drop of *Croton tig Q* in one ounce of cool water and let the patient take fast for 12 hours after taking this medicine. After four or five motions give the patient boiled rice and curd. If required, give a second dose after a long interval.

84. Carica Papaya Q 1x

It is very useful in indigestion, enlarged liver and spleen, pain in them after taking milk in the least quantity; yellowness of the conjunctiva; tongue coated white. Give *Carica 1x trit.* 3 grains one hour before and after meals.

3 seeds of *Carica* half an hour before and after meals cures indigestion and dyspepsia.

85. Cantharis Q

It stimulates and excites sexual organs in both sexes when 5 drops of Q internal thrice daily is used. Stop medicine after a week. If taken regularly for a long time it causes impetence.

86. Cimicifuga Q

It is a boon to despondent mothers who give birth to dead children only. Let the expectant mother take 5 drops of *Cimicifuga Q* once a day since the fifth month of pregnancy and she is sure to give birth to alive children. Aggravation of all complaints with the increase of menstrual flow. Give one drop every three hours.

87. Cod Liver Oil 1x Trit.

In marasmus, extreme emaciation, tissue waste give *Cod liver oil 1x* trit. 5 grains, thrice daily. In torpidity of liver and consequent night blindness alternate it with *Carduus marianus Q* 5 drops twice daily.

Mix one part of *cod liver oil* with nine parts of sugar of milk and get it be well triturated, and the 1x trituration is prepared.

88. Condurango Q

The moment there is suspicion of a tumour in the stomach having a cancerous tendency give *Condurango Q* 5 drops thrice daily and *Hydrastis Q* 5 drops twice daily to check further growth of tumour and cure it permanently.

89. China Q, 1x

It is an unique remedy in all ailments dependent on worms such as fever, derangements of stomach and bowels, epilepsy, tetanic spasms and convulsions unconsciousness; constant picking at nose, itching at the anus grinding of teeth in sleep, thick and whitish sediment in the urine; obstinate and irritable temperament and reveneous hunger call for the use of this drug.

burning debility and feeble pulse like *Arsenic* only lacking its restlessness. It is also beneficial in vertigo, pain in extremities, red eruptions with intense burning and fetid discharge from ulcers. Give 1x 2 drops or Q 5 drops every hour in emergency cases otherwise thrice daily.

51. Baryta Iod. Q

Acts on the lymphatic system, increases leucocytosis. Indurated glands, especially tonsils and breasts, tumefaction of carnical glands and stunted growth. Tumours. Quinsy To be given one grain thrice daily.

52 Beta Vulgaris 2x

It is of great service in chronic catarrhal states and tuberculosis. It is best adapted to pthisical patients. Children yield very rapidly to the action of this remedy. Use 2x tinct 1 grain thrice daily.

53. Betonica Q

It is very efficacious in pains in abdomen, hepatic region, transverse colon, in gall bladder, in right inguinal region and spermatic cords. Shooting pain in back of both wrist-joints Wrist drops. Give 5 drops thrice daily.

54. Boletus Taricis 1x

Very useful in quotidian intermittent fever. Chilliness along spine with frequent hot flashes, yawning and stretching during chill. Severe aching in shoulder and joints and small of back. Profuse perspiration at night with hectic chills and fever. Night sweat in pthisis. Give one drop thrice daily.

55. Blata Orientalis Q 1x

"Why should any patient of asthma die or suffer so long there is *Blata* in the phial ? *Blata* is unique remedy for asthma. During paroxysm of asthmatic dyspnoea first use *Passiflora incarnata Q* 60 drops mixed with *Blata orientalis Q* 10 drops in an ounce of hot water. This will act like a magic, suffocative dyspnoea will at once disappear and the patient will enjoy a sound and refreshing sleep. For a week repeat this process every night at bed time. In the day give *Blata Q* in 10 drop doses 4 times in an ounce of hot water, plus *Sulphur 6x* one dose early in the morning, continue this process for a week.

Then stop giving *Passiflora* and follow this course. *Bacillinum 200*, once in a week for a month *Sulphur 6x*, once in the morning. *Blata Q* 5 drops in an ounce of hot water thrice daily for a month. After a month follow this course. Stop giving *Sulphur*. Give *Bacillinun 1M*. once in a fortnight.

Psorinum 200 once in a week. *Blata 3x* in one drop doses thrice daily. Continue this process for a month. Then only *Blata 6* twice daily and *Bacillinum 1M*, once in a week. This is the process of the writer of this book based on his personal experiment and experience.

This process is mostly suitable in corpulent, sanguine and fat patients. In tubercular patients having asthmatic dyspnoea, *Blata* will relieve.

56. Blumia Odorata Q 1x

It is successefully used in bleeding piles, dysentery with

bloody stools and bleeding from uterus in gushes after abortion when all other remedies have failed.

In cough dry, barking, sawing croup with wheezing sound, aphonia and hoarseness it is of great service after failure of all remedies. Give *Blumia Q* in 5 drop doses 4 time a day, then 1x in 1 drop doses 3 times a day, with an ounce of cool water.

57. Boerrhavia Diffusa Q 1x

It is a very beneficial remedy in the following affections:—
"Attack of Beri-Beri and dropsy in every rainy season. Heaviness of feet with dropsy in feet, up to thigh. Patient cannot stand on account of sudden pain in lower extremities. Retention of urine, dribbling of urine with pain in the bladder, voilent palpitation of heart, of trembling and fluttering of heart, gasping for breath, aggravation of dyspnoea on physical exertion etc."

With these complaints *Borrhavia* is a great remedy in all kinds of dropsy. Give it in Q dilution 5 drops in cool water thrice daily for some time. After a few days give 1x in one dropdoses thrice daily.

58. Borrhavia Ripense 1x

It is similar to *Borrhavia diffusa* in all ailments and should be used in the same manner.

59. Berberis Aquifolia Q

It is chiefly useful in eruptions, scanty or pustular due to abnormality in the blood. Then use of this remedy removes morbidity and purifies blood and the skin affections gradually disappear in course of time. It cures promptly eczema of the head, scrotum and other parts, soothes excessive itching.

It is of much service in the eruptive stage of secondary syphilis and should be complimented with *Echinacea Q*, Both the remedies should be used in 5 drop doses twice daily in an ounce of cool water. It cures glanduler induration and chronic induration both of scrofulous and syphilitic origin. It stimulates all the glandular affections of the body, aids digestion and promotes general nutrition. It is also a tonic and corrective of hepatic disorders. It is a boon for young men and girls at puberty in checking formation of pimples and renders the skin smooth and soft.

Dose : 5 to 10 drop doses in an ounce of cool water 4 times a day.

60. Bryophyllum Calycinum Q

In the first stage of cholera, serious diarrhoea and dysentry with mucus or bloody stools, it is of great service. Give *Bryophyllum Q* 5 drops in an ounce of cool water after each stool in cholera, diarrhoea and dysentery and it will instantly cure the cases.

61. Bufo Rana Q

It is very efficacious in curing the habit of masturbation The patient always seeks a solitary place for masturbation. In epilepsy due to masturbation, attacks being only at night, *Bufo* acts as a magic. Give *Bufo Q*, 5 drops in an ounce of cool water twice daily and alternate it with *Oenanthe crocata Q*, in 5 dropdoses twice daily. In impotence due to masturbation it surpasses *Lyco, Phos* and *Agnus castus*. 5 dropdoses thrice

Give *Q* or 1x in one drop doses according to the emergency of the case.

90. Chininum Sulph 1x Trit.

It is a well nigh specific in ague with regular paroxysm of chill, heat and sweat. Give in 1x trit, 3 grs. a dose thrice daily before the paroxysms. It must be alternated with *Aconite nap 1x*, 1 drop a few minutes before the fixed time of chill and it will check ague more abruptly than all other known remedies.

91. Cedron

It is useful in all the diseases having the clock like regularity of the paroxysm especially in intermittent fever. It has been successfully used in malarial fever due to residing in a locality surrounded by stagnant water and marshy land with regular paroxysms of chill at a fixed hour ; chill and shivering with fever, scanty sweat or absence of sweat, congestion of blood in the head with or without bloody stools. Give *cedron 1x*, 1 rop thrice daily. In bloody dysdentery with ague alternate it with *Alstonia Q* 3 drops thrice daily.

92. Chionanthus Q

It gives instant relief and insures radical cure in gall-stone colic. Give *Chionanthus Q* 10 drops in an ounce of cool water every hour and oftener during paroxysm of pain.

To check the formation of stones and recurrence of pain give *chionanthus Q*, 5 drops thrice daily in an ounce of cool water and *carduus Q*, 5 drops in an ounce of cool water twice daily.

93. Cholestrinum 1x 2x

Dr. Swan of America has attained success beyond expectation in gall stone colic and Dr. Burnett of England has cured many patients of gall stone, colic in its various stages with medicine.

Give *Cholestrinum 1x* in 5 drop or 5 grains dose every half an hour or oftener during paroxysm of pain and give it in 2x trit or liquid, 1 gr. or 1 drop thrice daily for radical cure.

94. Caffein 1x Trit

Mix 1 part of *Caffein* with 9 parts of sugar of milk and get in well triturated' and the 1x trit is prepared. *Caffein* in 1x is a great heart stimulant ; Use it in cases of threatening heart failure due to frequent motions in 1 gr. dose over 10 to 15 minutes.

95. Chimaphilla Q 1x

It is a very beneficial remedy in chronic cystitis. Give its Q, 5 drops every three hours. It is a very beneficial remedy in violent pain, abscess and tumour of the breasts. Give Q, 5 drops thrice daily.

In abnormally dwindling and enlarged breasts give *Chimaphilla 1x* 1 drop thrice daily. Alternate it with *Mamary 3x* ; 2 tabs a dose thrice daily to restore the breasts to normal size, to make it firm, round, fleshy and light. Also *calcaria flour 3x* ; 5 grs. twice daily and *Alfalfa Q* one table spoonful after meals and see the result.

96. Clemats Q

In organic structure of urethra and consequent pain *Clematis Q* 3 drops every three hours acts like a magic. It is likewise a boon to swollen scrotum or testicles.

97. Cornus Acternifolia Q

Dr. Lutze suggests to give *Cornus Q* 5 drops thrice daily to check serous discharge from chilblains or broken skin and to cure it permanently.

98. Chloralum 2x Trit

It wonderfully cures recurring urticarial rashes. Give 2x trit, 2 grs. thrice daily.

99. Chlorate Hydrate 2x Trit

It is very beneficial in vomiting, diarrhoea, delirium, crop of boils, intense stinging pain in them due to sudden suppression of utricarial rashes.

It succeeds marvellously when *Apis* and *Urtica urens* fail to bring the case to normalcy. Give 2x trit, 2 grs. thrice daily.

100. Crocus Q

It has cured cancer in the last part of the large intestines.

Give Q 5 drops every three hours.

101. Chomocladia Q

It cures miraculously the white epidermis of lepsory, leucoderma. Give 5 drops thrice daily.

102. Crisophanic Acid Q

It is a very useful remedy in dandruff and reeling of the skin of palms. Give 3 drops thrice daily.

103. Ceasalpania Bondulosa-Quninia Indica-Nata.

It is regarded and used as a patent medicine in all kinds of ague and is more efficacious than quinine but never harmful like it.

Following are the characteristics of this drug :

"Flashes of heat like flaming fire in all stages of intermittent fever, amelioration from washing with cool water. Drops of sweat temporarily on face, neck, shoulders and chest. Great debility during prodermal stage ; lies muttering with closed eyes.

Pain in the enlarged liver and spleen before paroxysm of lever.".

It matters little whether these characteristic symptoms are present or not *Quinia indica* cures all kinds of malarial fever more promptly than other remedies. Tincture 5 drops thrice daily.

104. Calotropis Gigantia 1x

Calotropis gigantia is possessed of great virtue in purifying blood and is very efficacious in curing syphilis in all its stages, leprosy in feet, around nails, fingures etc. in all kinds of putrid gangrenous ulcers and leprosy are associated with intense, intolerable burning, violent burning in the whole of alimentary canal. Likewise it has been used with marked efficacy in asthma dependent on syphilitic virus or mercurial poisoning.

In these affections give *Calotropis 1x* 1 drop thrice daily and alternate it with *Echinacea 1x* 3 drops twice daily.

Calotropis is likewise very efficacious in curing intermittent fever due to malaria or kalaazar with enlarged spleen and liver.

Following are the characteristics of the intermittent fever :

"Chilliness prominent in the intermittent fever, chilliness and shivering start from feet and ascend upward through spinal cord. Chilliness relieved by heat of fire, and worse by motion. Heat in the face and head with coldness in the body.

Flashes of heat on cheeks as if burning with fire, sweat alternating with chilliness. Vertigo and delirium are the concomitants. In these affections give *Calotropis 1x* 2 drops four times a day.

105. Calotropis Lactum 1x, 2x

It is more efficacious and acts more promptly than *Calotropis gigantia* in all its characteristics. Moreover its efficacy has been proved in vomiting, watery diarrhoea, toothache, enlargement of spleen and many forms of skin diseases.

1x, 2x, 1 gr. or 1 drop thrice daily.

106. Clerodendron Infortunata Q, 1x

It is very useful in worms of children with foamy, watery, diarrhoeic stools and water brash.

In chronic intermittent fever it is very beneficial with enlargement of liver and spleen, slight fever in the after noon, loss of appetite, constipation, indigestion, nausea and water brash.

Tincture 5 drops or 1x, 2 drops thrice daily.

107. Cephalenra Indica Q, 1x

It is very beneficial in chronic malaria, dysentery and skin diseases. It is very efficacious in dysentry with mucus and blood, green stools with pain in navel region when other remedy have failed.

In chronic malaria it is of great service with intense burning in palms, soles, face and eyes. It is very beneficial in intolerable burning in palms and soles due to excess of bile headache, due to bile and sun stroke.

Tincture 5 drops or 1x, 2 drops thrice daily.

108. Coleus Aromaticus Q, 1x

It acts principally on kidneys. It is very useful in suppression and also retention of urine due to inactivity of the kidneys and bladder, with pain in the right kidney burning pain during and after micturition.

It is very beneficial remedy in gonorrhoea, nephritis and cystistis with discharge of mucus membranes, deposit of red sand in the urine and haematuria.

Give *Coleus* Q, 10 to 15 drops or, 1x, 2 drops every fifteen minutes or thrice daily according to the case.

109. Cyndon Dactylone Q 1x

It is an important remedy in curing haemorrhage from any orifice of the body such as haematuria, hemoptysis, haemorrhage from lungs while coughing, haemorrhage from uterus, menorrhagia and bleeding from piles.

Give *Cyndon dactylone* Q, 5 drops every three hours and alternate with *Gerarium maculatum* Q, 10 drops thrice daily. When some relief is obtained give the 1x of both, 2 drops in the same manner.

It is also useful in retention of urine and painful micturition. It is an important remedy in secondary syphilis and should be alternated with *Calotropis lactum*. It should be used with success in chronic dysentery with fever, general or local dropsical affections.

Dose : Q in 5 drops or 1x in 2 drops every three hours, then thrice daily.

110. Caulophyllum Q, 1x

It has proved to be very beneficial in false labour. It is very efficacious in the following symptoms :

"Labour pains weak and deficient, foetus does not pass downward. Rigidity of organs. Pains are deficient during labour, patient is exhausted and fretful. Spasmodic rigidity of os, delaying labour, pains like needles in cervix. Pains become weak ; flagging from long protracted labour, causing exhaustion ; thirsty, feverish ; tormenting useless pains in the beginning of labour."

Give *Caulophyllum* Q 5 drops every 10 to 15 minutes. If malposition of the foetus is ascertained, first give a dose of *Pulsatilla 200*. It will correct the position of the foetus, then give *Caulophyllum* as directed above and see the magic.

Caulophyllum is likewise beneficial in abortion.

"Habitual abortion from uterine debility. Threatening abortion, spasmodic bearing down pains. Passive haemorrhage after abortion." In such cases give *Caulophyllum* Q, 5 drops every 10 to 15 minutes and alternate it with *Trillium 3x* 2 drops every 10 to 15 minutes.

Caulophyllum is likewise successfully used in spasmodic dysmenorrhoea, with scanty flow. Give *Caulophyllun* Q 5 drops, *Xanthoxyllum* Q 5 drops and *Abroma Radix* Q 5 drops alternately at intervals of half an hour. And for radical cure all these remedies should be used in 1x potency 2 drops each once a day.

In prolapsus uteri when the uterus is retroverted or prolapsed due to defective nutrition with little or no local congestion, give *Caulophyllum 1x* 2 drops thrice daily. In climacteric disorders give *Caulo. 3x*; when there is great tension, unrest, indisposition to work and worry about trifles. It is especially useful in rheumatism of the phalangeal and metacarpal joints in females. Give *Caulophyllum 1x* 1 drop 4 times a day in rheumatism.

111. Desmodium Gingeticum Q, 1x

It is useful in intermittent fever. Chill at 7 A. M., continues for two hours. Intense burning in palms, soles, eyes and face since the commencement of heat. Slight perspiration on forehead, hand and feet just after the chill is over. Headache as if tightly bandaged.

Give Q 5 drops or 1x 2 drops thrice daily.

112. Damiana Q

Damiana invigorates the nervous system and increases the tone of body. It is serviceable in cases of exhaustion from physical exertion and mental over-work.

It controls chronic prostatic discharge. It cures incontinence of urine in old people by strengthening the spinal nerves.

It cures spermatorrhoea in weak exhausted subjects. Its principal use is for the cure of impotency in both sexes whether caused by injury to the spine, sexual excesses, gonorhoea or syphilis.

Generally it is given 2 to 4 drops in an ounce of cool water 3 to 4 times a day.

In impotency give *Damiana Q* 5 drops twice daily, *Avena*

sativa Q 5 drops twice daily and *Aswagandha* Q 5 drops twice daily if it is due to sexual excesses.

If impotence is due to injury to the spinal nerves, give *Damiana* Q 5 drops twice daily and *Hypericum* 1x 1 drop twice daily.

If impotence is caused by syphilis and gonorrhoea give *Damiana* Q 5 drops twice daily and *Agnus castus* 1x 2 drops twice daily.

The second method is to give *Damiana* Q 5 drops, *Salix nigra* Q 5 drops and *Saw palmetto* Q 5 drops each once a day in an ounce of cool water in impotency due to any cause.

113. Dioscorea Q

It affords prompt relief and affects a radical cure in gall stone colic where there is relief in colic by standing erect or bending backward. Dr. Burt says that the grand sphere for the use of *Dioscorea* is among necrosis of the bowels and stomach where the iliac and umbilical plexus are in a state of great hyperaesthesia, the pain and spasms being unbearable ; and the author adds that the pains force patient to bend double though it makes him worse and there is relief by standing erect or bending-backward.

With this last characteristic *Dioscorea* is amazingly curative in biliary colic, flatulent colic, flatulent dyspepsia and gastralgia. Give *Discorea* Q 5 drops every 10 to 15 minutes.

114. Drosera Q, 1x

Drosera is the most important remedy in whooping cough with the following symptoms :

"Paroxysms of cough follow each other so violently that

he is scarcely able to get his breath. Crawling in larynx provoking cough. sensation as if some soft substance were there in the larynx, with sticking extending to right side of pharynx. Paroxysms of cough from tickling in larynx frequent, ending in gaging, vomiting and cold sweat, usually worse at night immediately after lying down or after midnight."

Give *Drosera Q*, 2 to 5 drops or 1x, 1 drop. Never give a second dose immediately after the first : it will not only prevent the good effect of the former but would be injurious. If needed give the second dose at the time of paroxysm in the next night.

I have cured a case of enlarged spleen associated with whooping cough of *Drosera* type with this remedy.

A case of whooping cough was cured by the author by *Drosera* associated with whooping cough of the above nature. *Drosera 200* is specific for goitre.

115. Dulcamara 1x, 2x

It is found useful for colic and diarrhoea following suppression of an eruption in cold weather. *Dulcamara* cures that form of Bright's disease following scarlet fever or from malaria ; specially related to very sensitive bleeding ulcers with granulation, phagedenic ulcers. It is suitable in inflammatory rheumatism due to suppressed perspiration induced by change from a high to low temperature or from cold wet weather. It suits those colds that have a sluggish circulation of the brain with trembling and chilliness as if in the bones. It is a reliable remedy in threatening paralysis of lungs especially in the bronchitis of old people and young children. It is also recommended in slighter form of nym-

DULCAMARA

phomania when associated with heat, itching and herpetic eruptions about the genitals. It is useful in salivation of mercury which is notably worse in damp weather. It is a very valuable remedy for the cough of old people worse from change of weather to cold and wet. It is very frequently useful in bronchial catarrh with free greenish expectoration. It is of great service in lameness of the small of back or stiffness across the neck and shoulders, servere drawing pains in muscles of back with fever after getting cold or wet. It is wonderfully useful in diarrhoea at the close of summer, hot days and cool nights with changeable stool.

Give 1x or 2x in one drop doses every 3 hours or thrice daily according to the nature of the case.

116. Eupatorium Perfoliatum Q, 1x

It has proved to be great beneficial in ague with the following symptoms :

"Intermittent fever, chill 7 to 9 A.M., intense aching in all bones before chill, soreness in bones, bruised feeling everywhere preventing lying in bed and causing despair, moaning and crying out, inability to lie on the let side ; vomiting of bile between chill and heat insatiable thirst before and during chill and fever, periodicity third or seventh day"

Give *Eupatorium Q*, 5 drops or 1x, 2 drops every 15 minutes during paroxysm of fever and 4 times during prodormal stage.

117. Eupatorium Ayapan Q, 1x, 2x

It is a very efficacious remedy in snake-bite like *Echinacea* and *Lucus aspera*. Its internal as well as external use saves life from snake-bite.

It is very useful in bleeding from lungs with cough in consumption, in bleeding from bowels in dysentery due to ulcer therein and cures white coloured ulcers.

In pulmonary haemorrhage give *Eupatorium ayapan 2x* 1 drop 4 times a day; give 1x 1 drop thrice daily in dysentery; Q 5 drops every 10 to 15 minutes in snakebites. Give 1 drop in ulcers. Mix; 1 part of Q with 1 part of glycerine or olive oil for external use in ulcers. Plain mother tincture to be rubbed on injury due to snake-bite.

118. Euphorbium 1x, 2x

It is useful in gastro-intestinal irritation; chronic diarrhoea when accompanied with cerebral irritation and delirium. It has been used topically for cancer and has cured epithelioma, gangrene, pustular and eczematous eruptions.

Give *Euphorbium 1x* one drop every half an hour in severe diarrhoea and 1 drop thrice daily in other affections.

119. Euphorbia Pilulifera Q

It is a specific remedy in all kinds of asthma and it has cured desperate cases of asthma. Give tincture 10 drops 10 minutes apart during paroxysm and thrice daily when paroxysm is over.

120. Euphrasia Q, 1x

It is very efficacious remedy in acute eye-affections. Profuse, bland, fluent coryza and excoriating lachrimation. Traumatic conjunctivitis, blepharitis, corneal ulcers." It has been successfully used to remove spots, vesicles, ulcers on cornea—

Rheumatic iritis; iris reacts tardily to light; acous humour cloudy, burning, stinging pains worse at night, acrid lachrimation. Clarke says: "As an eye-lotion *Euphrasia* has great value. I have seen corneal opacities removed by it."

In the opinion of the author it is useless to kill time and patience of the patient by using other drugs in the treatment of opthalmia and conjunctivitis. One can solely depend on *Euphrasia* in inflammatery condition of the eyes.

Give *Euphrasia 1*, one drop every two hours or four times a day according to the severity of the case. Mix one part of *Eupharasia* Q with nine parts of rose water 3 drops three to four times a day should be instilled into the eyes with the aid of dropper. When a child does not progress in class due to his defective brain, give *Euphrasia* Q 5 drops thrice daily and in course of time the child will head the list of top ranking students.

121. Embelia Ribens 1x, Q

Embelia ribens is a very beneficial remedy in all abnormalities dependent on worms especially in children. It is useful in indigestion, diarrhoea, fever, starting and frightful shrills in sleep, grinding of teeth etc. Q 10 drops every 3 hours and a fasting for 24 hours.

Then 5 drops thrice daily.

122. Echinacea Angustifolia Q

Echinacea acts as an effective anti-dote to all kinds of poisons and thereby cures all diseases caused by them.

It is most reliable remedy in snake-bite, dog-bite, poisonous thorns, fish-bones, oyster and other shells. In these case the wound should be washed with soap and water and covered with a piece of cloth constantly kept moist with a solution of *Echinacea* 1 part with three parts of water.

Internally *Echinacea* should be used frequently 10 drops every half an hour or oftener in an ounce of water, less frequently later.

The medicine diluted with equal parts of boiled water may also be injected hypodermically at the site of snake-bite for immediate action of the medicine. In stings of insects and scorpion, pure mother tincture may be rubbed on the site of sting and it will instantly relieve pain and prevent inflammation. It is marvellously valuable in curing syphilis in all its stages. Hypodermic injection of *Echinacea* will hasten the purification of blood from syphilitic virus and then remove permanently all the manifestations produced by this virus. Give *Echinacea* Q, 10 drops 4 times a day internally with an ounce of water. Mix equal parts of *Echinacea* with olive oil or glycerine and apply externally on syphilitic ulcer, chancre, buboes and eruptions. In syphilitic affections of the mouth, gargles prepared by mixing 1 part of *Echinacea* with 9 parts of water should be used.

In gonorrhoea give *Echincea* Q 10 drops 3 times a day and *Vesicaria com.* Q, 10 draps, 3 times a day in an ounce of water. The vagina may be packed with gause saturated with a lotion 1 in 9 and the same lotion may be injected in the urethra in male and female alike.

It is of great service in the last stage of external cancer for the pain. Use it internally, externally and hypodermically.

ECHINACEA ANGUSTIFOLIA

It acts as a magic in malignant, foul smelling wounds and gangrenous ulcers due to injury and other causes. It will save life and limbs and do away with the necessity of amputations. Inject *Echinacea* Q, hypodermically every other day. Give it internally in 10 drops doses 4 times a day. Apply an ointment of *Echinacea* Q prepared by equal part of glycerine.

In septic poisoning caused by absorption of germs from wounds, in puerperal fever, puerperal septicaemia, pelvic cellulitis and septic peritonitis its action is marvellous. Temerature rapidly falls with disappearance of all other symptoms.

Give *Echinacea* Q, 10 drops in an ounce of hot water every hour or every 2 hours internally. Inject it hypodermically every 12 hours. Use locally as a douche for vagina and tampon saturated with it (equal parts of glycerine and *Echinacea* Q may be applied to the cervix uteri.

In boils and carbuncles, eczema of any kind, ulcers, in scrofulous ulcerations and affections of glands in Psoriasis and in all forms of skin diseases, it is a most important remedy. It cures the local manifestations and at the same time corrects the blood impurity, thereby preventing recurrence.

Give *Echinacea* 1x 1 drop 4 times a day. Use ointment of *Echinacea* Q 1 in 4 parts of glycerine or compresses 1 in 9 parts of hot water. It is of great service in erysipelas. By the use of this drug, burning disappears, extension of the disease is checked and fever subsides.

Give hypodermic injections of *Echinacea* Q every 6 hours. Give *Echinacea* 10 drops every 2 hours. Use externally the compresses of *Echinacea* Q 1 part mixed with 9 parts of hot water.

In cerebro-spinal meningitis cold compresses of the lotion of this drug should be used. Internally give it every 2 hours in 5 to 10 drop doses. Also use the indicated remedy alternately.

In foul diarrhoea, in malignant dysentery, cholera infantum, it likewise acts like a magic, and is an effective intestinal disinfectant.

Give 2 to 5 drops in an ounce of cool water 4 times a day and inject it into the bowels, 20 drops of the tincture with 4 oz. of warm water.

In typhoid fever it strongly acts as an anti-septic on the intestines and as a tonic. The stools diminish in frequency and the fetid odour disappears. The course of the fever is checked and sustained. Give *Echinacea* Q 3 drops every 2 hours internally with an ounce of cool water. Also inject it hypodermically. Besides this to cure give *Baptisia* Q 10 drops 6 times daily and a single does of *Typhoidine 200*. In delirium and insomnia of typhoid fever, give 60 drops of *Passiflora incarnata* Q in an ounce of hot water at 8 P M. and repeat the same dose at 9. P. M. or at any hour of the day when urgently required, espcially in violent delirium.

123. Esculentine

Esculentine is of great service in promptly reducing fat like *phytoline* and it is a harmless and an agreeable medicine, It has asserted its merits as an antifat in the practice of a large number of physicians. Like *Phytoline* it reduces bulk and converts flabby, fatty tissue into healthy muscular tissue. Simultaneously it strengthens the heart and improves the general health. It also controls and cures the intolerable rheumatic pain to which the obese is subject.

Give one table spoonful of *Esculentine* Q in an onuce of hot water and *Phytoline* Q, one table spoonful, each twice daily before meals.

Fatty and starchy food should be taken in moderation.

124. Eueslyptus Globe Q

Dr. Dewie Boericke and Antsuz advise to use this drug in intermittent fever of malarial origin in absence of any distinct symptoms.

High temperature, violent palpitation of heart, expectoration of phlegm mixed with pus and mucus, digestive disorders, fetid odour of the stools, nephritis, lassitude and blood sepsis, call for the use of this drug Q 3 drops every 3 hours.

In inflammation of the kidneys give this drug Q 2 drops every 2-3 hours.

125. Equisetum Q

It cures the habit of wetting the bed when *Sepia, Causticum*, etc. fail

Tincture 3 drops thrice daily. Grinding of teeth, boring and picking at nose-due to worms after failure of *Cina* and *Santonine* with very offensive, red and dirty urine.

Give 1x, 2 drops thrice daily.

126. Ficcus Religiosa Q, 1x

It is very efficacious in haemorrhage of bright, red, blood, from any orific of body such as metrorrhagia, menorrhagia haemoptysis, haematuria, haemorrhage from lungs, bowels vicarious menstruation. Give Q, 5 drops or 1x 2 drops every 10 to 15 minutes or four times a day according to the nature of the case.

127. Ficcus Indica Q, 1x

It is successfully serviceable in profuse mucus and blood in acute dysenteric stools ; emission of blood followed by evacuation of faccus with colic and tenosmus forcing the patient to bend double.

It is very useful in long lasting, profuse haemorrhage of bright, red blood, frequently at short intervals from uterus.

It is very efficacious in spermatorrhoea due to excessive seminal loss. It is likewise curative in genorrhoea and diabetes with haematuria and burning during micturition.

Give Q, 5 drops or 1x, 2 drops 4 times a day with an ounce of cool water.

128. Ferrum Phos 2x

Ferrum phos maintains the equilibrium in circulatory system and aids in equal distribution of blood in every cell and tissue. Hence, it is very useful in anaemia due to loss of blood or any disease ; haemorrhage from any orifice of the body. Bleeding due to cuts or injury is promptly controlled by this remedy.

It is likewise useful in congestion and hyperaemia and ailments associated with them.

In bleeding give *Ferrum phos 2x* 5 grs. every 10 to 15 minutes or oftener as required.

In profuse bleeding due to extraction of tooth, wash the mouth with hot water. Put 10 grs. of *Ferrum phos 2x* in cotton and put it in the bleeding part and press hard. Do this twice or thrice every 15 minutes. Simultaneously boil

10 grs. of *Ferrum phos 2x* in 2 c. c. of plain water, get it cooled and inject it hypodermically on the upper and outer quadrant of any arm. In bleeding due to cuts or injury clean the site injured with water, put 5 to 10 grs. of *Ferrum phos 2x* on the injured part and press it. One application is more than sufficient.

If the vein is cut or torn do like this twice or thrice and tie hard above and below the site. Let the patient take *Ferrum phos 2x* 5 grs. every 10 to 15 minutes or if the case be very serious inject hypodermically as described above.

In the excessive bleeding from any orifice same measure can be adopted except the external application.

In ordinary cases, it should be given every 2 hours or 4 times a day.

129. Fluid Cerefolius Q

It is of service in nephritis, cystitis and enlargement of the prostatic glands. Bright's disease, renal dropsy, prostatitis, particularly in old men. It is dieuretic, soothing and antiseptic. It has a powerful tonic influence upon the sympathetic nerves and soil is of great value in sexual debility especially of a neuraesthenic origin.

Give half to one tea-spoonful of this drug in an ounce of water every 3 hours or 4 times a day.

130. Fraximus Americana Q

In enlargement of the uterus this wonderful remedy will often reduce it to normal size preventing the necessity of an operation and the organs will gravitate back into the correct position.

Uterine tumours, fibrous growths, and distressing backache are cured by this medicine. Give this drug 5 to 10 drops in an ounce of water 3 to 4 times a day.

131. Fucus Vesiculous Q

Fucus contains a large proportion of *Iodine* and is a powerful remedy for the reduction of obesity. It increases the rapidity of digestion and diminishes flatulence.

Give 5 drops of the tincture twice daily for a long time for reduction of fat. Alternate it with *Phyloline* Q 5 drops twice a day.

132. Fluid Calendula Q, 1x

It is a great anti-septic remedy and can be safely used in all kinds of septic-gangrenous conditions. In the last stage of pox when septic condition threatens life, it is of great value.

Give *Calendula 1x*, 2 drops every three hours and alternate it with *Echinacea* **Q** 5 drops thrice daily in all septic and gangrenous states.

133. Geranium Maculatum Q

It is the most valuable remedy for controlling haemorrhage. It succeeds magically when all other styptics have failed.

In bleeding from lungs and stomach give it 1 tea-spoonful with an ounce of hot water every 15 to 30 minutes till the bleeding is checked. Afterwards give 10 drops, 3 to 4 times a day to prevent recurrence.

Besides controlling haemoptysis in cansumptives, it also moderates nocturnal perspiration and teasing cough, and checks diarrhoea. In post-partum haemorrhage, *Geranium* is valuable. It is also valuable in metrorrhagia and leucorrhoea. Give *Geranium Q* 5 drops 4 times a day and also injections into the vagina with a lotion of 1 part of *Geranium Q* + 9 parts of water should be given.

In bleeding from intestines and kidneys give 10 to 20 minims every 3 hour to ensure better results.

For piles and prolapsus of the rectum give *Geranium Q* 5 drops thrice daily and also use it externally mixed with equal part of olive oil or glycerine.

In epistaxis give *Geraninm Q* 1/2 dr. in an ounce of water every hour or 2 hours as the case may be and simultaneously tincture pure or diluted with water in the ratio of 1 : 9 should be syringed into the nasal cavity or a cotton wool tempon saturated with the tincture should be introduced into the nostrils.

The tincture should be injected on the nasal polipi once a day, the tumours will shrink and fall off after a few days.

Geranium should be applied on chronic ulcers either pure or mixed with olive oil or coconut oil one in ten.

It should be used externally in the same manner in bedsores. It strengthens the tissues and promotes prompt healing.

134. Gallium Aparine Q

It is of great service in cancer. Give tincture 30 to 60 drops mixed with milk four times a day and see the miracle.

135. Gelsemium Q, 1x

It is of great service in the following diseases :

1. Deafness resulting from abuse of quinine-*Allen*.

2. Nueralgic rheumatism with soreness of muscles as if bruised—*Cowperthwaite.*

3. Specially useful in paralysis when affecting single group of muscles more especially about the mouth, eyes throat, larynx, chest, extremities and sphincter—*Cowperthwaite.*

4. It is our most valuable remedy in post-diphtheritic paralysis.—*Farrington.*

5. It is an admirable remedy for the premonitory stages in puerperal convulsions.—*Farrington.*

6. It is an excellent remedy in the lying in room ; false labour pains ; pains shoot up instead of bearing down ; there is an atomic condition, the os widely dilated ; pain insufficient or entirely absent ; rigid os ; severe after pains. Puerperal convulsions and twitchings—*Cowperthwaite.*

Give Q, 5 drops, or 1x, 2 drops every 15 minutes in emergency cases and thrice daily in other cases.

136. Glonoine 2x, 3x

It is of great service in the following affections :

1. It is very efficacious in insanity caused by long continued exposure to heat of the sun ; the patient thinks he is Lord Almighty.—*Allen.*

2. In angina pectoris with fluttering of the heart and violent beating as if it would burst; the chest feels open, with labored breathing, pains radiating in all directions even into arms with loss of power in the arm.—***Allen.***

3. For the simple determination of blood to the head which sometimes proceeds apoplexy, it is very effective, and also for that which often occurs in softening and tumours of the brain.

4. In threatened apoplexy and when apoplexy has taken place if the violent pressure keeps on, think of this remedy.—*Kent*

5. A most valuable remedy for affects of sun-stroke, a rapid and efficient remedy.—*Allen* and *Richard Hughes.*

6. One of the best remedies we have for the congestive form of puerperal convulsions—that from which is announced by rush of blood to the head, especially if there is albuminuria.—*Farrington.*

7. Shocks in brain synchronous with pulse.

8. Cerebral congestion or alternate congestion of head and heart. Brain feels too large, full bursting ; blood seems to be pumped upward ; throbs at every jar, step.

9. Intense congestion of brain from delayed or suppressed menses, headache in place of menses with glowing redness of the face.

10. Put 10 drops of *Glonoine 2x, 3x* or *3x*, in 4 oz. water and give a tea spoonful every hour or 4 times a day according to the nature of the case.

137. Grindalia Q

This remedy is indicated in chronic bronchial asthma and

chronic spasmodic bronchial cough when they are attended with profuse, tenacious expectoration and relief from expectoration. The breath stops when the patient goes to sleep and awakes with a start, gasping for breath.

Give *Grindalia Q*, 5 drops every 15 minutes during paroxysm and thrice daily in normal state.

138 Guaiacum Q

It is useful in chronic rheumatism of the upper extremities and in lumbago especially after abuse of mercury or dependent on syphilis.

It is employed in the treatment of secondary syphilis and contraction of affected parts. Numbness of all limbs. Immovable stiffness of contracted limbs. It is indicated in stiffness and dryness of the throat. Underwood says that it is specially valuable in follicular tonsillitis, rheumatic pharyngitis and tonsillitis when there is violent burning in throat. It is said to relieve extremely offensive expectoration in Phthisis.

Q, 1x, 2 drops in an ounce of water, thrice daily.

139. Gynocardia Odorata — Chalmongra Q

It is very beneficial remedy in leprosy, secondary Syphilis, rheumatism, gout, psoriasis, eczema, scabies and other cutaneous eruptions.

Give *Chalmongra Q*, 2 drops or 1x, 1 drop thrice daily. Its external application causes asthma and other chronic affections.

140. Hamamelis Q

It is an important venous remedy. It has a specific relation to venous troubles, venous congestions, haemorrhages, vericose veins and haemorrhoids.

It is regarded as the *Aconite* of veins—veneous congestions, vericositis of every kind, venous haemorrhages. It is useful in bad effects from bleeding; prostration out of porportion to amount of blood lost.

It is a very efficacious remedy in piles—bleeding profusely with burning, soreness, fulness and weight in back as if it would break on urging to stool, itching at anus.

Give Tincture 5 to 10 drops, 15 minutes or oftener, or 3 times a day.

141. Helleborus Niger Q 1x

It is of great service in meningitis—acute cerebro-spinal, tubercular with exudation and cephalic cry. Rolls head day and night. Bores head into pillow. A condition of sensorial depression, sees, hears, tastes imperfectly; general muscular weakness which may go on to complete paralysis, accompanied by dropsical effusion.

It is very beneficial in dropsy of brain, chest, abdomen, after scarlatina, intermittents.

It is of great service in concussion of brain after *Arnica* has failed. Concussion with extreme coldness of the body, except head or occiput which may be hot.

Greedily swallows cold water, spoon but remains unconscious, chewing motion of the mouth.

Dr. Phillips states that he gets excellent results in post-scarlatinal dropsy with 10 drops doses of the tincture.

In other cases 1x. in 2 drop-doses should be given, every 3 hours.

142. Helonias Dioica Q

It is a great uterine tonric. Loss of sexual desire and power with or without sterility. Profound melancholy, deep depression with a sensation of soreness in the womb; a consciousness of womb. Prolapsus uteri and ulceration of cervix and a constant dark fetid bloody discharge, after parturition, face shallow; pain in small of back with great vaginal irritation. It is of great service in excessive uterine haemorrhage. Prolapsus of uterus, leucorrhoea; os protrudes externally.

Uterus low down, fundus tilted forward. Prolapse from atony.

Threatened abortion, especially in habitual abortion. Albuminuria during pregnancy.

Nipples sensitive, tender, painful; breasts swollen; intolerable to pressure of cloth.

Headache and anaemia with uterine derangements. Tired backache in females.

5 drops of Tincture thrice daily for a longer time.

143. Hydrastis Q

It is successfully used in cancer and pre-cancerous states, before ulceration when pain is the principal symptom.

In those suffering from cancer it has given a degree of relief and improved the general health and while it may have no influence over the cancerous dyscrasia but a little over

HYDRASTIS

scirrhous tumours developing in glandular tissue. Goitre of puberty and during pregnancy.

Give *Hydrastis Q*, 5 drops thrice daily in cancer of the soft palate. Give *Hydrastis 1x*, 2 drops every 3 hours in cancer of the last part of large intestine.

When *Arsenic* fails in cancer with intense burning, *Hydrastis* Q has proved to be very beneficial in 5 drop-doses, 4 times a day and if the cancer is external also apply continuously a lotion of this medicine Q. 1 in 9 parts of pure water.

It is very beneficial in putrid tumours when used Q, 5 drops thrice daily and also external application of Q, 1 part + *olive oil* 3 parts is essential. *Hydrastis Q*, 5 drops thrice daily is very efficacious in loss of appetite, in cancerous and phthisical patients.

Dr. Allen advises to give it to increase weight in patients who have been cured from tuberculosis by *Tuberculinum*.

Hydrastis is a very beneficial remedy in nasal polipy when there is discharge of watery yellowish green acrid and excoriating substance, ulcer in septum, accumulation of phlegm or mucus in fauces.

Gonorrhoea, thick yellow discharge. Debility after spermatorrhoea.

Leucorrhoea tenacious, ropy, thick, yellow, ulcer in cervix and vaginae. Pruritus vulva.

Stomatitis in nursing women, especially ofter abuse of mercury or chlorate of potash.

Constipation with haemorrhoids. It is useful in constipation that is dependent on inertia or congestion of the lower abdomen or when it is the result of sedentary habit or purgative medicines; during pregnancy; after parturition.

Gall-stone colic with jaundice. Ulceration of rectum. Prolapsus of rectum.

It is successfully employed in ulceration of skin, fissured nipples, indolent ulcers, lupus, eczema and leprosy during the ulcerative stage.

A patent medicine for habitual constipation, may be alternated with *Carduus marianus 3x*.

Dose : For constipation give Q, five minims in water before breakfast and it is highly satisfactory. In other cases give 5 drops of Tincture 3 to 4 times a day.

144. Hydrocotyle Asiatica Q, 1x

It is an important remedy in leprosy, elephantiasis, syphilitic effections, granular cancer of uterus.

Dr. Ardont used it with much success in granular ulceration of wombs and in pruritus vaginae.

Great thickness of epidermoid layer of skin and exfoliations in scales. Psoriasis in trunk, extremities, palms and soles. Erysipelatus redness. Red spots. Circular spots with scaly edges. Dry eruptions. Erythema on face, neck, back, chest, arms, thighs with much itching, with copious sweat.

Miliary eruptions on neck, back. chest; pricking and itching on different parts. Intolerable itching, specially of soles. Bruised feeling in all muscles. Wandering pains in muscles of chest and legs.

Give Tincture 5 drop doses or 1x. 2 drop doses thrice daily.

145. Hydrocyanic Acid 1x, 2x

It extricates one from the jaws of death in the stage of collapse when extinction of life seems inevitable.

Cyanosis, collapse due to some pulmonary condition, not a cardiac collapse, the patient gasps for a longer time as if this is the last attempt.

In this stage give *Hydrocyanic acid* 2x, 2 drops every 3 to 5 minutes on the tongue and a few drops on the face and forehead. When condition improves stop medicine or if needed give on longer intervals.

This remedy is indicated in diseases of the cerebro-spinal nervous system that appear suddenly and with great severity.

Angina pectoris. Whooping cough. Paralysis of lungs. Cyanosis. Coldness within and without. Great prostration.

Give 1x in one drop doses.

146. Hypericum Q

It is useful in injury of nervous tissue, spinal injury, shocks and concussions, also in spinal irritation, in punctured wounds, lacerated wounds and gun-shot wounds.

It is a very valuable remedy to remove pain following surgical operation especially amputations, lock-jaw temporary or permanent after amputation.

Excessive pain and soreness of the affected parts. Violent pain and inability to work or stoop after a fall on the coccyx, can not walk from affection of spine. Feeling of weakness and trembling of all the limbs. Numbness and crawling in the limbs, hand and feet.

Give Tincture in 5 drop doses at intervals of 10, 15 or 30 minutes in emergency cases. In other cases 3 to 4 times a day.

In chronic lock-jaw after amputation 200 or higher potencies should be tried if Q is not sufficient.

147. Hymosa Q

It is the most effective remedy in the treatment of rheumatism and rheumatic fever. It quickly brings down the fever, diminishes pain and cures the inflammation of the joints.

It prevents disease of the heart in rheumatic fever. It is very efficacious in acute and chronic arthritic and muscular rheumatism. It relieves the pain and removes the virus from the system thereby prevents recurrence.

In gout it neutralises the acidity of the blood, removes deposits from joints and cures all disorders due to the disease.

It cures lumbago rapidly. In neutralgias acute or chronic in any part of the body, facial, intercoastal, ovarian, uterine, it is a certain remedy. It marvellously cures sciatica.

It cures instantly rheumatic tonsillitis, rheumatic iritis, etc. It has no injurious effect on heart or kidneys. It frees the system from uric acid diathesis and is beneficial in lucomotor ataxia.

Give *Hymosa Q*, 1 dram and *Passiflora incarnata Q*, 1 dram in 2 oz. of hot water followed by plenty of hot water or soda water. Repeat the same after an hour. Then *Hymosa Q* alone, 1 dram in an ounce of hot water, followed by a heavy draught of hot water or soda water, every 3 hours in acute stages.

In chronic cases *Hymosa Q*, 1 dram in an ounce of hot water, followed by plenty of hot water or soda water, 4 times a day is sufficient.

148. Helarrhena or Chenomorha Anti-dysenterica Kurchi Q

It is a very efficacious remedy in all kinds of acute and chronic dysentery.

It affords instant relief and radical cure in acute and chronic dysentery with great debility, prostration, loss of appetite when all other well indicated remedies have failed. Frequent twisting pain around navel at short intervals, relief of pain after evacuation of mucus and blood ; aggravation after lying on right side.

Give it Q, 5 drops every 2 hours and alternate it with *Aegal marmelus Q*, 20 drops in an ounce of cool water every 2 hours in acute dysentery. In chronic cases give *Helarrhena* 1x, 3 drops, 4 times a day.

149. Hygrophilla spinosa Q, 1x

It is a very beneficial remedy in leprosy and deep ulcers after putridity of blood.

Small eruptions and red blisters like measles and redness of skin about eruptions exudation of scanty bluish fluid after itching.

In these effections give *Hydrophilla Q*, 5 drops thrice daily.

Paroxysms of intermittent fever at 10-11 A.M. Appearance

of urticarial rashes with intense itching during heat, aggravation from heat and amelioration from cold applications.

In these affections give 1x, 2 drops every three hours.

150. Hemidesmus Indica Q, 1x

It is a very efficacious remedy in curing all diseases dependent on blood poisoning as it renders the blood free from septic conditions.

It has cured eruptions due to abuse of mercury.

Dr. E. J. Browning recommends this medicine in syphilis, syphititic eruptions, syphilitic arthritic pains, indigestion and loss of appetite and says that it can be substituted for *Sarsaparilla*.

Give Q, 5 drops or 1x, 2 drops thrice daily.

151. Hydrophobin 3x

It removes hydrophobia instantly after biting of mad dog, cat or jackal.

Give *Hydrophobin 3x*, 2 drops, 4 times a day and alternate it with *Echinacea* Q, 5 drops thrice daily.

After some time give a single dose of *Hydrophobin 200*.

152. Jacaranda Caroba Q, 1x

It is of great service in gout and rheumatism of joints and right thigh due to syphilis and sycosis. It is also useful in warts and redness after the syphilitic ulcer is cured.

It is very efficacious in the priapism of penis with heat and pain in it without any urinary trouble.

It is very effective in ulcer, swelling and phymosis of the

crepuce and discharge of pus from beneath it after drawing it upward.

Ttncture in 5 drop doses thrice daily.

153. Jatropha Curcas 1x, 1

"Stools like rice-water pass like gunbullets with vomiting of watery substance, spasms in extremities and coldness of whole body with relief from sinking hand in water," are the characteristics of this most effective drug.

Give 1x or 1 in 1 drop doses every 15 to 30 minutes.

154. Justicia Adhatoda Q, 1x

It has gained universal reputation for curing many catarrhal conditions of the respiratory system. It is a great expectorant and soothes teasing cough in coryza, pneumonea, bronchitis, phthisis and clears the lungs.

Following are the characteristics of this most beneficial drug.—"Aphonia, gagging after coughing, wheezing sound in the throat expectoration of thick yellow phlegm streaked with blood, incessant violent cough ; accumulation of abundant phlegm with little or no expectoration on coughing ; loss of power of smell and taste with frontal headache ; discharge of thick, yellow phlegm mixed with blood in violent nocturnal dry cough with going and wheezing."

It is very beneficial in the first stage of phthisis and all kinds of pulmonary diseases with discharge of blood in the phlegm. Likewise it is very effective in whooping cough of children with gagging after coughing, stiffness of body, face cyanotic and constipation.

Give 3 drops of Q or 1 drop of 1x, 4 times a day.

155. Justicia Rubrum 1x

It is a successful remedy in profuse haemoptysis, and haemorrhage from lungs during paroxyms of cough in phthisical patients. It is more affective than *Justicia adhatoda* in these troubles.

Give Q, 3 drops or 1x, 2 drops, 4 times a day.

156. Jaborandi 1x, 2x

It is a very effective remedy in profuse debilitating sweat in phthisis.

Use 1x or 2x, 2 drops, 4 times a day to relieve sweat.

157: Kalmegh Q, 1x

It is a very famous remedy in kala-azar, malaria and in intermittent fever with double paroxysm. Chill at 8-9 A.M. or 10-12 o'clock. Alternating states, alternations of chill and burning; sometimes amelioration from cold application and sometimes aversion to it. Chronic malaria and kala-azar or infants with enlargement of infantile liver, yellow eyes. White coated tongue; constipation, stools acanty and black; burning in palms and soles.

Its specific action is on liver especially in children. Jaundice of infants with yellow urine; infantile liver, enlargement of liver and spleen with pain in them.

Give 2 to 5 drops of mother tincture or one drop of 1x, 4 times a day.

158. Lufa Bindal Q, 1x

Its main action is on the spleen and liver. It is more efficacious than *Ceanothus* and acts better than it in splenic troubles, such as splenitis, enlargement of spleen and liver.

Give Q, 5 to 10 drops twice daily and *Ceanothus Q*, 5 drops twice daily.

It is of great service in gall-stones and other biliary affections.

Give *Lufa bindal Q*, 5 drops twice daily and *Carduus Q*, 5 drops twice daily.

It is externally applicable in piles.

Mix 1 part of *Lufa bindal Q* with 1 part *olive oil* and apply on the piles.

159. Lufa Amara or Fuetida Q, 1x

It is a very efficacious remedy in intermittent fever with chill in the morning, thirst, headache, vomiting and diarrhoea, pain in spleen and liver.

It abruptly checks vomiting and diarrhoea when *Ipecac* fails.

Give Q, 5 drops thrice daily in intermittent fever and 1x, 1 drop, a dose after each stool and vomiting.

160. Leucus Aspera Q, 1x

It is said to be of great service in snake-bite in all its stages It may be inhaled when patient has lost the power of swallowing; may be taken internally Q, 5 drops every 10 to 15 minutes. Externally it should be applied on the site of bite.

It is likewise efficacious like *Echinacea* in stings of scorpion and other poisonous insects.

It should be rubbed on the affected parts.

In chronic malaria with enlargement of liver and spleen, it is very efficacious. It arouses appetite in convalescents after malaria or any kind of fever.

In these affections give Q, 5 drops or 1x, 1 drop thrice daily.

161. Lathyrus Sativus Q, 1x

It is a very efficacious remedy in beri-beri, paralysis of lower extremities and dropsy.

The patient cannot put his legs on right place, both teh knees clash together with emaciation of the lower extremities and muscles behind them. Feet turn blue and swell on hanging them. Heels and toes cannot be lifted from ground due to violent spasms and convulsions.

Always drowsy and yawning.

Give Q, 5 drops or 1x 2 drops thrice daily.

162. Labelia Inflata Q, 1x

It is very efficacions in vomiting of pregnancy with violen nausea, morning sickness, cold sweat on face, chronic complaint of vomiting of profuse mucus and great prostration after vomiting.

Headache with nausea and vomiting with great lassitude worse after tobacoo chewing and its smoke, aggr, after noon.

Dysponoea even after slight cold, increased respiration with decreases of pain in asthma.

Over-sensitivenoess in lower spina, has to bend forward for fear of contact with both.

163. Laurocerasus 1x

On sudden onset of apoplexy give *Laurocerasus* 1x, 2 drops every hour.

It will arrest the further progress of the disease and cure it instantly.

164. Makaradhwaj 1x

It is a great cardiac, mental, nervous and seminal tonic with violent palpitation of heart, other vulva or effections, indigestion vertigo etc. and is more efficacious than *Carbo veg,* and *Kali, phos.*

It quickly stimulates the systems in convalescents after long lasting diseases.

It is also valuable in spasmodic cough and asthma with aggravation at night and a checking sensation during paroxysm of asthma.

Give 1x, 2 drops every 10 to 15 minutes in emergency cases otherwise thrice daily.

165 Menispernum 1x

Incessant flow of uterine heamorrhage with bright red. clotted blood, aggravation from motion or movement.

Menorrhagia and untimely metrorrhagia of bright red-blood.

Give 1x, every hour, 2 drops a doses.

Then thrice daily.

166. Mutha Q, 1x

It is a great tonic to digestive system. It is very efficacious in indigestion, dyspepsia, acidity, diarrhoea, flatulence, etc.

5 drops of tincture 4 times a day or 2 drops of 1x, 4 times a day.

167. Mica 1x, 2x

It has proved to be great beneficial in debility due to

excessive loss of blood and vital fluids; nervous debility, impotence, phthisis, diabetes and chronic fevers.

1x, 1 drop or 2x, 1 drop 4 times a day.

168. Momordica cherentia Q, 1x

High temperature due to undeveloped small-pox, measles. It aids the appearance of eurruptions, and thus cures the patient.

Watery discharges from eyes and nose with cough, nausea, constipation or diarrhoea.

Give Q, 5 drops every 4 hours if associated with constipation, and 1x, 2 drops with diarrhoea.

169. Mullen Oil Q

Its internal use is of great service in incontinence of urine, wetting the bed at night. Constant dribbling of urine or frequent urging to urinate.

2 drops of Q, 4 times a day.

170. Nyctanthus Arbortriotis Q, 1x

It is very efficacious in bilious fever with vomiting and purging of bile or constipations; insatiable thirst before chill; vomiting of bile just after drinking; nausea in all stages of fever; thick, white or yellow coating on the tongue.

Thick, white coating on tongue with constipation and thick, yellow coating with bilious diarrhoea is the characteristic of this drug.

Pain in liver, stitching pain in hepatic region on pressure with deep red urine.

Give 1x, 1 drop, 4 times a day.

172. Natrum Murbit Q, 1x

It is possessed of all the virtues of *Natrum mur.* but is more efficacious than the latter.

Paroxysm of chill at 10-11 **A.M.** Headache indicates the fast approaching chill. Violent chill and shivering, intense thirst, headache with stupefaction, blue lips and nails. Intense pain during heat, vomiting with headache, amelioration of all symptoms after perspiration. Stinging pain in liver and spleen in prodromal stage. Spots and scales on tongue, blisters on lips. Strong desire for salty and spiced things and aversion to bread.

173. Nufer Leuteum 1x

It is an unique and wonderful remedy in all kinds of seminal and nervous disorders, such as nocturnal emissions, early ejaculation, impotence, relaxation and looseness of genitals, thinness of semen and neuraesthenia dependent on them.

1x 2 drops 4 times a day.

174. Malaria Officinalis 1x

It is very efficacious in bringing down the high temperature of malarial intermittent fever. Give this medicine 1x, 2 drops every half an hour or oftener and the temperature will become normal very soon without any untoward consequences.

In malarial cachexia suppressed by quinine it is a very marvellous remedy. It removes the bad effects of abuse of *Quinine*. The suppressed intermittent fever, especially of low marshy land, appears in its real form is cured.

Give 1x 2 drops 4 times a day. Afterwards give 1M. 1 dose.

175. Manganise Dioxide

It is very efficacious in amenorrhoea due to evacuing and consumption. It cures all these diseases and causes free menstrual flow. Give Q, 1 grain 4 times a day.

176. Nux Juglans Q, 1x

It is a very efficacious remedy in consumption with the following symptoms : "Cough, aphonia ; heaviness in chest, distention and hardness of abdomen, diarrhoea, indigestion, glandular swelling with pus in axilla and its vicinity. It radically cures acne in young girls at puberty.

Give *Nux juglans* Q or 1x 2 drops 4 time a day.

177. Nux Vomica Q, 1x

In the very commencement of tetanus *Nux vomica* Q or 1x in 2 drops doses promptly arrests the progress of the case and cures it.

178. Oldenlandia Herbacea Q, 1x

It is very efficacious in acute and chronic malaria with fever after exposure to cold ; headache, burning in palms, soles and eyes, intense thirst, bilious diarrhoea, yellow coating on tongue ; one day the paroxysm is very mild and the next day it is very severe.

Q 5 drops or 1x, 2 drops 4 times a day.

179. Oenanthe Crocata Q

It is very efficacious for the treatment of epilepsy and epileptiform convulsions, acute and chronic.

2 drops of tincture in an ounce of cool water.

180. Ocimum Sanctum Q, 1x

It is of great service in intermittent fever. Constantly yawning and stretching during chill, spasms in extremities, violent electric-like shocks in nerves, violent internal and external chill and shivering. Thirst increased, with the rise of temperature, flashes of heat from face, eyes and mouth. Scanty sweat in axilla, neck, shoulders and chest.

It is very efficacious in the first stage of consumption with slight fever, distressing dry cough, expectoration of phlegm streaked with blood. In dyspnoea of children and old men the patient cannot lie, nor to sit down.

Tincture, 5 drops or 1x, 2 drops 4 times a day.

181. Ova Testa 3x.

It is the most important remedy for leucorrhoea profuse and offensive with sensation as if the back were broken into two and tied with a string.

It controls haemorrhage from the uterus and has cured cases of cancer of os uteri. 1 grain of 3x 4 times a day.

182 Origanum Q, 1x

Its main action is on the nervous system. It is a very efficacious remedy in voluptuous dreams, nocturnal emissions, excessive strong desire for sexual intercourse and their evil consequences.

Tincture 5 drops or 1x, 2 drops thrice daily.

183. Pas Avena Q

It instantly relieves any kind of pain or colic. At the same time it maintains neural equilibrium. It is very useful remedy in headache, neuralgia, sciatica, grippe, abdominal or ovarian colic. Give Q, one tea-spoonful in an ounce of hot water followed by a draught of plenty of hot water, every 15 to 30 minutes.

In hysteria, insomnia, convulsions and all degrees of nervousness, it acts like a magic. Thrice daily as directed above.

184. Passiflora Compound Q

It is one of the best nerve sedative. It is very wonderfully useful in all conditions resulting from impaired nerve functions and so is invaluable in insomnia, convulsions, epilepsy, tetanus, chorea, paralysis agitans, locomotor ataxia, in spasmodic and non-spasmodic asthma.

It is most valuable remedy in convulsions of childhood and epilepsy. All nervous disorders due to derangement of the genito-urinary system are amenable to it.

15 drops to 1 dr. every 15 minutes or thrice daily.

185. Passiflora Incarnata Q

It is the most reliable remedy in insomnia due to pain and inflammatory conditions in acute diseases.

In tetanus, give 1 dr. in an ounce of hot water every 15 minutes, then every 3 hours.

In epilepsy, give 1 dram dose of it with an ounce of hot water at bed time and alternate it with *Oenanthe crocata Q*, 5 drops twice daily.

In rheumatism gout and sciatica, it aids the action of *Hymosa* and other remedies and induces sleep.

In meningitis it pacifies the mental troubles and induces sleep. In delirium tremens it acts like a magic In all forms of mania, it lessens the mental excitement and gradully cures the disease. It may be safely used in alternation with the well-selected remedy.

In painful menstruation, unbearable labour pains, prolonged labour, eclumpsia during labour, after pains etc. it affords great and instant relief.

In hysteric affections and a peculiar spasmodic cough of young unmarried girls it is very beneficial.

In asthma give a tea-spoonful of this medicine and it acts like a magic. Give *Blata orientale Q*, 5 drops thrice daily and a dose of *Passiflora incarnata Q*, 1 dr. at bed time in an ounce of hot water.

It diminishes the craving for alcohol in drunkards and cures drinking habit if used in alternation with *Spiritus caladium quersus* Q. Give each medicines 10 minims twice daily in milk or tea.

In delirium of typhoid, give 1 dram in an ounce of hot water every hour till it induces sleep.

186. Prerero Brena Q

It is very beneficial in renal colic, difficult micturition with strong urging for urination, fulness in bladder, violent pain in bladder and back, crying bitterly due to pain strangury. red sand or brick-dust in the urine, give Q, 30 drops in 2 oz. of hot water every half an hour.

187. Phytoline Q

It is a fat-reducer. It reduces fat, makes the muscles thiner, more firm and stronger. The patient looks considerably younger. Difficulty in walking, sitting, palpitation and dyspnoea on least exertion, nausea and eructation, disappears slowly and steadily. It corrects the fatty condition of the heart and liver and cures rheumatism and gout associated with obesity. It also removes sterility inobese subjects and enables them to be fortunate mothers.

Bowels should be kept regular by occasional use of enema cr laxatives.

2 drops in an ounce of hot water, 4 times a day.

188 Pulsatilla Q

In amenorrhoea *i.e.* stoppage of menses due to any cause give *Pulsatilla Q*, 5 drops thrice daily, and the menses will appear after a short period.

189. Recinus Communis Q, 1x

It is very efficacious in suppression of milk with amenorrhoea and its use promotes secretion and increase of milk with commencement of menstrual flow. External application and massage of *Q*, in breasts stimulates the secreting power of mammary glands and adds the increase and flow of milk in abundance.

Internally give 1x, 2 drops thrice daily.

190. Ranwolfia Serpentina Q, 1x

It is the most important remedy to cure high blood pressure.

Give 5 to 10 drops of the tincture twice daily in the beginning, then give 1x, 1 drop thrice daily.

It is very efficacious in violent form of insanity and

madness. It controls the cerebrum and central nervous system instantly and the patient becomes normal very soon.

Give 1x, 2 drops 4 times a day. If associated with menstrual disorders also give *Asoka* 1x, 2 drops thrice daily.

191. Ruta Q

It is very efficacious in gangrenous tumour or cancer of the uterus. Give Q 5 drops thrice daily.

192. Symphoricarpus Recemosa Q

It is a specific remedy to check morning sickness and distressing vomiting of pregnancy.

Give Q, 5 drops thrice daily.

193. Spiritus Glandium Quercus Q

It is a very powerful medicine in diminishing craving for alcoholic drinks and it can be safely used for a long time.

Give 10 drops of Q in tea or milk twice daily and 10 drops of *Passiflora incarnata* Q in milk or tea twice daily.

194. Succus Amogara Q

It is a specific in all stages of syphilis and septicaemia.

In boils, carbuncles, abscesses, diphtheria and typhoid conditions, it is a marvelleous remedy and purifies the blood.

Give in 1 dram doses of Q, thrice daily and alternate it with *Echinacea* Q, 5 drops twice daily.

Use lotions of Q 1 in 9 of water externally.

195. Syzygium Jambolinum Q

It is the most important remedy of universal fame in curing diabetes mellitus. It promptly diminishes the quantity of sugar and frequency of micturition.

It also cures ulcers and carbuncles dependent on diabetes with high specific gravity in urine, with intense thirst, and debility.

It also cures intense heat in upper parts of body, small and red blisters with itching, intense thirst with or without fever.

Use Q, 5 drops, 4 times a day.

196. Solanum Xanthocarpum Q, 1x

It acts like a magic in all kinds of aphonia on failure of well selected remedies.

It is very efficacious in colds and coryza, cough, pneumonea, bronchitis, dry cough, with aphonia and in asthmatic dyspnoea.

In acute fever it is likewise beneficial with burning thirst, vomiting, cough, loss of appetite and pain in ribs.

It is also very beneficial in gall bladder and urinary troubles such as retention of urine etc.

Give Q, 5 drops or 1x, 1 drop every 3 hours.

197. Secale Cor Q

It acts like a magic in amenorrhoea due to any cause with intense burning and great longing for cold things in weak, delicate subjects. First ascertain whether she is pregnant if the patient is pregnant in her first, second or third month, do not use this drug, otherwise it will cause abortion.

Give Q, 10 drops thrice daily.

If by mistake abortion has been affected by use of this drug, *Secale cor.* 200, 1 dose will check the tendency of uterine haemorrhage.

198. Strophanthus Q

Like *Passiflora incarnata* and *Spritus glandinum quercus Q*, it also is very efficacious in dimishing the craving for spiritus liquors, slowly and surely.

Give Q, 10 drops thrice daily.

199. Symphytum Q

It is very efficacious in curing cancer due to injury or cancer of the breasts and chest.

Give Q, 10 drops 4 times a day.

200. Saw Palenetto Q

It acts mainly on the prostatic gland of the old people.

It is very useful in frequent painful micturitions, inflammation of the bladder, insomnia due to frequent urging for micturition at night.

It diminishes the size of prostate and cures ailments associated with it

It is a very beneficial remedy in hydrocele and spermatorrhoea.

It is a marvellous remedy to cure impotence and sexual inertia in both sexes.

Give Q, 10 drops thrice daily.

201. Santonine 1x

Dr. Custis recommends *Santonine 1x* in all kinds of worms in 2 to 5 grains doses every 3 hours.

In my opinion the best way to use *Santonine 1x* is as follows :—

Give *Santonine 1*x, 2 grs., 4 doses in a day and *Castor oil* drops in an ounce of cool water at bed time. Repeat this every third day for a fortnight.

After a fortnight give a dose of *Cina 200*.

202. Stigmata Medius Q

Says Dr. Hausen, "It is a very beneficial medicine for intolerable pain during passing of gall-stones if given Q, 20 drops every 10 to 15 minutes."

203. Sebal Serrulata Q

It is very efficacious remedy in impotency and loss of power of expulsion of urine due to enlargement of prostatic gland.

Give Q, 5 drops every 3 hours or thrice daily.

204. Spongia Q

According to Dr. Persey, any kind of skin disease is cured by *Spongia Q*, 2 drops, thrice daily.

205. Salix Nigra Q

It is a great sexual tonic for males. It cures nocturnal emissions, spermatorrhoea and impotence.

It cures ovarian pain before and during menses, nervous disorders and leucorrhoea.

Give Q, 10 drops thrice daily.

206. Senega Q.

Its action on the respiratory system is well marked "cough dry and teasing, wheezing sound, opperssion in the chest, constriction in the chest, accumulation and rattling of abundant sputa with dyspnoea, aphonia aggr. lying and walking, amel, bending head and on perspiration" are the guiding symptoms for the use of this drug.

Give Q, 5 drops, 4 times a day.

207. Strychnia Phos 2x, 3x

It is a very beneficial medicine in paralysis. In acute stage give 2x, 3 drops every one or 2 hours. In chronic stage 3x, thrice daily.

208. Saracenia Q

It removes the spots and fills up the pits of smallpox in acute stage.

Give Q, 3 drops thrice daily.

In chronic pits of smallpox *Variolinum C.M.* once in a month is a spicific measure to fill the pits.

209. Sulphur Q

It is a very efficacious remedy in all kinds of amenorrhoea with intense general and local burning, amel. cold applications; aversion to bathing, craving for open air.

Give Q, 5 drops 4 times a day.

Warning: Do not give it in stoppage of nausea in early months of pregnancy or it will abort it.

210. Cimicio Q

It is very effective in delayed first menstruation in puberty and youth or irregular menses.

Give Q, 5 drops, 4 times a day.

Alternate with *Asoka 1x*, 1 drop twice daily.

211. Tinospora Cordifolia 1x

It is very efficacious in chronic malaria, especially after abuse of *Quinine* with enlarged spleen and liver, yellowness of conjunctiva, diarrhoea and vomiting. In acute malaria, there is burning in soles and palms. extreme mailaise, heaviness and tearing in extremities before paroxysm of chill. Temperature mild. Chilliness at about 4-5 P.M. Thirst during heat followed by perspiration, associated with digestive disorders.

Give 1x, 2 drops, thrice daily.

212. Thymol 1x

Its main action is on the genito-urinary system and is very useful in nocturnal emissions with voluptuous dreams, frequent priapism, prostatic discharge during micturition with burning pain in lumbar region, restlessness and prostration, aggr. after mental and physical exertions.

Give 1x, 1 drop thrice daily.

213. Trichosanthes Disica Q, 1x

It is a very beneficial remedy in cholera when there are frequent watery stools, vomiting, thirst, burning everywhere, restlessness, great prostration, perspiration, extremities cold, pulse weak or imperceptible.

It is very efficacious in irregular paroxysms of intermittent fever; chill at 10-11 A.M, 2-3 P.M. and 6-9 P.M. with vomiting of bile, thirst, vertigo, vomiting as soon as the water is drunk. It resembles *Arsenic alb.* and should be alternated with it in irregularity and alternation of shotes.

It is very efficacious in amenorrhoea of long lasting duration.

Give Q, 30 drops, thrice daily.

214. Tribulus Terrestris Q, 1x

It is very beneficial in impotency, gonorrhoea and mental, nervous and physical weakness.

Give Q, 5 drops thrice daily.

215. Thlapsi Bursa Pastoris Q

It is very efficacious in haematuria, renal colic and dropsy due to kidney affections.

Give Q, 5 drops every hour or thrice daily.

216. Thyroidine 3x

It is a specific remedy in serofula, mental inertia and physical awkwardness due to undeveloped or retarded functions of thyroid gland.

Exostosis of the bones of face and extremities and affections due to excessive activity of the pituitary glands are amenable to this marvellous drug.

Give 3x, 5 grs., thrice daily and alternate it with *Hekla lava 3x*, 2 grs., twice daily.

217. Trillium 3x

It is a specific medicine to cheak bleeding of abortion very quickly.

Give 3x, 2 drops every 15 minutes.

218. Tathelin 1x Trit, Q. Trit

It promotes quick development and growth of the body.

Give Q trit or 1x trit, 2 grs. thrice daily.

219. Vesicaria Communis Q

It is a specific remedy to cure gonorrhoea, acute and chronic, gleet. It checks the progress of the disease and permanently eliminates the virus from the system.

It cures inflammation of urethra and bladder due to gonorrhoea and prevents formation of stones in the bladder.

It promptly relieves the renal colic, eliminates stones and checks formation of the same permanently.

It prevents uric acid diathesis. It controls the suppurative stage of urethra due to T.B. or gonorrhoea.

It relieves the inflammation of kidneys, increases the quantity of urine and cures dropsy due to renal disorders.

It promotes discharge of urine when it is suppressed or retained due to any cause.

Give Q, 10 drops every hour in emergency cases and 5 drops every 3 hours in ordinary cases.

220. Viburnum Opulus Q

It is very beneficial in spasmodic dysmenorrhoea; pain in the legs of expectant mothers, false labour pain and post-partum pains.

It prevents habitual abortion and pre-mature delivery.

It corrects leucorrhoea following menstrual flow, violent uterine pain.

Give Q, 10 drops every half an hour, otherwise 5 drops thrice daily.

221. Viburnum Prunifolium Q

Its main action is on the uterus and is very beneficial in uterine haemorrhage and dysmenorrhoea. It promptly corrects the morning sickness of pregnancy. It diminishes the violence of labour pain and makes its bearable. It controls the post-partum haemorrhage. It has a great power to save the tendency of habitual abortion and miscarriage. If an attempt has been made for abortion or miscarriage by dint of a powerful poisonous drug it removes the bad effects of the drug and protects the embryo by preventing abortion and miscarriage. It turns sterile woman in lucky mothers by regulating and stengthening the power of conception and delivery. Give Q, ten drops every hour in emergency cases and five drops thrice daily in ordinary cases.

222. Vaccininum Metallicum Q

It is very efficatious in gangrenous stage of intestines in dysentery. It controls the situation and cures disentery.

Give Q, 10 drops thrice daily.

223. Viscum Album Q

It is very efficacious in gonorrhoeal rheumatism of join' and glands, especially in woman.

Give Q, 5 drops thrice day.

224. Valeriana Q

It is very beneficial in chlorosis with nervous disorders or hysteria.

Give Q, 5 drops, thrice daily for a long time.

225. Zincum Valeriana 3x

It cures promptly the neuralgic pain of ovaries, according to Dr. Ludlam.

Give 3x, 2 drops thrice daily every 3 hours.

CHAPTER II

EXTERNAL MOTHER TINCTURE

External mother tinctures can be used in the forms of oil, ointment, lotion and liniment with great efficacy in relieving the pains and distress of the patients whereas internal mother tinctures act into cure the diseases.

Method of Preparation

(1) Lotion is prepared by mixing 1 part of Q external, in 9 part of hot water.

(2) Oil is prepared by mixing Q external, 1 part with 9 parts of olive oil or glycerine.

(3) Ointment is prepared by mixing 1 part of Q external with 9 parts of white vaseline.

(4) Liniment is prepared by mixing 1 part of Q external, with 9 parts of hot water + 10 parts of olive oil.

Lotion can be used in abrasions of skin due to cut, flow, bruises, etc

Ointment should be applied in old wounds and ulcers to heal them promptly.

Liniment should be rubbed in pains in chest. Oils should be used in inflammatory pains and swellings.

1. Acid Carbolic Q external

It relieves inflammation of ears by dropping some drops of this external medicine by mixing 5 drops of *Carbolic acid* in 1 dram of Glycerine.

Mix *Carbolic acid* 1 dram + Glycerine 1 oz + distilled water 5 oz. Put a few drops in ears. It changes the ears having fetid otorrhoea and removes the foeter.

In gangrenous eczema in external ears, wash it with the lotion of *Carbolic acid* and apply pure olive oil.

It removes offensive odour of the mouth by washing it with the carbolic lotion.

Great success has been gained in scales ; burns and ervsipelas by applying the lotion and ointment of *Carbolic acid*.

2. Aesculus Hip. Q Ext.

Lotion and ointment of this drug are very beneficial in curing piles.

3. Aconite Nap Q Ext.

It is very beneficial drug in acute neuralgia and inflammation. Lotion should be used in inflammation whereas ointment should be used in neuralgic pains.

4. Agaricus Q Ext.

Application of its lotion and ointment is very beneficial in chilblains and fissures of winter.

5. Apis Mel Q Ext.

It is very beneficial in stings of bees and wasps when applied pure external Mother tincture with cotton.

6. Argentum Nit Q. 200

Mix 3 drops *Argentum nit 6* ext. with $\frac{1}{2}$ oz. of water and it will quickly relieve acute ophthalmia. In chronic cases put 1 drop of *Arg-nit 200* in one dram of water and use a few drops thrice daily.

7. Acid Benzoic Q Ext.

Its lotion is very beneficial in inflammation of the veins and nerves of ligaments. Mix *Benzoic acid*, Q 15 drs + rectified spirit 3 drs. + distilled water 8 oz. and wash the affected part.

8. Arnica Mont. Q Ext.

Its lotion and ointment are very beneficial in cuts, sprains, abrasions, bruises, bed-sores and strains, etc.

In iritis due to blow, the application of lotion Q external and internal use of *Arnica 3* promptly cures it.

When cattle has been injured, apply the lotion and ointment of *Arnica* Q external.

9. Badiaga Q Ext.

Its ointment or oil is very beneficial in swelling of glands,

10. Belladonna Q Ext.

It is wonderfully effective in sore throat; hoarseness of voice; hard, dry cough; redness of the inflamed parts and abdominal pains. Application and rubbing of the oil or ointment is advised in these complaints.

In abscess or boils inside ears, give hot compresses, followed by 2 drops of *Belladonna* Q external, every 2 hours.

It will abort or hasten suppuration and relieve the pain.

In peritonitis rub its oil on the abdomen and it will relieve all the disorders at once.

11. Berberis Vulgaris Q Ext.

In abdominal colic its internal and external use has proved very efficacious.

Rub Q Ext. in form of oil.

12. Bellis Perenis Q Ext.

It affords great relief in wounds and ulcers due to injury. Apply its oil.

Apply its oil on moles and they will disappear.

13. Bryonia Alb Q Ext.

In rheumatic stiffneck, sciatica, pain and hardness of joints, rub its oil very gently. In pain of chest rub its liniment

14. Calendula Q, Ext.

It is used as a safe dressing in any catarrhal and inflammatory conditions of the mucus membranes.

Its internal use and external use in the form of lotion, oil and ointment are very efficacious in ulcers and wounds caused by blow, injury, cuts and burns.

Its lotion is everywhere beneficial even in ulcers inside the pelvic region, rectum or in external syphilitic or cancerous ulcers.

15. Cantharis Q Ext.

Its internal use in 3rd potency and external use in the form of lotion are very, efficacious in burns with anything. It soothes the burning and pain due to burns. Afterwards use its ointment to cure the ulcers caused by burns.

16. Causticum Q Ext.

Like *Cantharis* it is also very useful in burns especially in after effect of burns if used internally in 6th potency and externally its ointment.

17. Capsicum Q Ext.

Its oil is very efficacious in inflammations with burning as if someone has applied pepper.

18. Carduus Q Ext.

Its lotion, oil and compresses are very efficacious in all complaints of liver whatever name be given to the ailment.

19. Cinereria Maritima Succus Q Ext.

It is successfully used to cure cataract, corneal opacities and spots. It has proved more beneficial in the beginning of cataract and has saved many from surrendering to knife.

It absorbs the remnants in the eyes even after operation.

It cures all kinds of ulcers in eyes. For radical cure *Cinereria* at least one ounce should be used.

Put 3 drops in each eye thrice daily and let the patient remain lying with closed eyes at least for 10 minutes after instillation of the medicine.

20. Chloride of Zinc Q Ext.

In spasm of urethra during pregnancy wash the vagina with a lotion of this drug. Mix 1 grain of this drug with 1 oz. of water and the lotion is prepared.

Simultaneously the internal use of *Spigelia 6* and *Staphisagria 6* in alternation, 2 doses each is recommended.

21. Euphrasia Q Ext.

Its external use is very beneficial in all kinds of opthalmia, redness and violent pains. Mix *Euphrasia Q ext.* 1 part + 9 parts of rose water. Instil 3 drops in each eyes every 2 hours, later on thrice daily.

22. Mullen Oil Q

It is specific remedy in all ailments of ears. It is of the greatest significance in deafness of any kind.

In all affections in the ear, neuralgic or inflammatory, *Mullen oil* is the remedy.

In pain and swelling of external ear paint it.

Its application about the induration and enlargement of lymphatic glands is highly recommended.

In all complaints of ears, put 3 drops of *Mullen oil* in each ear every 3 hours, then thrice daily.

In orchitis or in inflammation of the testicles mix 30 drops of *Mullen oil* in an ounce of *Olive oil* and rub on the affected part.

It promptly relieves the teasing cough, aphonia and hoarseness of voice if rubbed gently in the chest in *Bronchitis, Pharyngitis* and *Phthisis*.

Mix 1 part of *Mullen oil* with 2 parts of *Olive oil* and rub the throat and chest.

Mix 30 drops of *Mullen oil* in an ounce of *Olive oil* and inject in urethra to relieve the inflammation and pain therein.

In inflammation and ulcer of cervix-uteri, apply this remedy with the aid of cotton tempon.

23. Plantago Major Q

In pains of any kind in teeth and gums apply this remedy 4 times a day with cotton and see the miracle.

24. Phytolacca Q

Paint pure *Phytolacca Q* in the inflamed, indurated glands of any place, specially of neck, face, tonsils and breasts. It can be used in form of compress also. For this mix 1 part of ext. with 9 parts of hot water.

25. Ruta Q Ext.

Its ointment is very beneficial in tumours according to Dr. Cooper.

In ulcerative tumour, sprinkle *Iodoform 1x trit.* or *Carbo veg 2x trit* with grand success.

26. Rhus Tox Q Ext.

Its oil should be succussfully rubbed in rheumatism of joints, lower part of the back, sprains, strains in wrist, tendons and muscles.

27. Silicea Q

All kinds of supperative abrcesses and boils apply the lotion of *Silicea Q* and you need not use a lancet for evacuation of pus.

28. Symphytum Q Ext.

In fractures and complaints of injured cartilagaes mix 1 part of *Symphytum Q* with 5 parts of hot water and use it as compress.

29. Styrax Balsam Q Ext.

Apply pure *Styrax balsam Q ext.* in scabies dry or moist once a day and wash it with soap and hot water 12 hours after the application for 4 days and all scabies shall disappear without any untoward result.

30. Shookum Chuck Q Ext.

Mix. 1 part of this drug with 3 parts of *Olive oil* and apply in all kinds of eczema with marvellous effect.

31 Sulphur Q Ext.

In all kinds of itching and scabies paint this oil *i.e.* 1 part of *Sulphur Q ext.*+9 parts of *Olive oil* twice daily.

32. Tamus Communis Q Ext.

Its oil or ointment should be applied in all kinds of chilblains and bruises, trauma.

33. Tenereum Q Ext.

In polypus of nose inject its lotion in the affected nostril and the polipi will shrink soon.

In polipi of other parts apply its oil.

34. Thuja Q Ext.

In warts, especially soft ones and ingrowing toe-nails apply pure *Thuja ext.* or its oil.

35. Urtica Urens Q Ext.

In burns of any part apply pure drug or its lotion without water : Also use $3x$ internally.

36. Veratrum Viride Q Ext.

Rubbing of its oil in rheumatic swelling to afford prompt relief.

CHAPTER III

THERAPEUTIC HINTS

Abortion—Blumia odorata, Corpus tenterum, Cimicifuga, Helonias, Trillium.

Amenorrhoea—Asoka, Secale, Pulsatilla, Sulphur.

Asthma—Blata orientalis, Passiflora inc., Canabis sat., Maka-radhwaj, Senega.

Acne—Kali-brome., Nux ; Juglans.

Anaemia—Fer. phos.

Apoplexy—Laurocerasus.

Bleeding Piles—Blumia odorata.

Bleeding from Lungs—Acalypha ind., Ficcus religiosa, Blumia odorata, Hamamelis, Cyndon dactylon, Justicia rubrum, Occinum, sanctum, Eupatorium ayapan.

Beri-beri—Lathyrus, China.

Bubo—Bufo rana.

Cholera—Camphor. Coffea mocha, Recinus, Trychosanthis, Dioca.

Chlorosis—Abroma Augusta, osoka, Corpus tenterum.

Coryza—Camphor, Occinum.

Collapse—Camphor, Hydrocyanic acid, Aconite nap., Aconite radix, Kali cyanatum, Zinc cyanide, Caffein.

Chorea—Agaricus, Nux vom, Pas avena.

Cough—Abroma, Cyndon dactylon, Justisia adhatodea, Jastisia rubrum.

Constipation—Abroma augusta, Castor oil, Azadirecta Indica, Audersonia, Croton tig.

Diarrhoea—Achirenthus Camphor, Chaparo amar, Josa, Mutha.

Dysentery—Alstonia, Aegle marvelos, Castor oil, Cephalendra indica, Helarena, Anti-Dysenterica.

Dysmenorrhoea—Abroma augusta, Abroma radix, Xanthoxyllum, Asoka, Corpus leuteum, Cimicifuga.

Diphtheria—Acenasia, Echinacea.

Diabetes—Abroma augusta, Syzygium jambolinum.

Dyspepsia—Aquaphychota, Caricopapaya.

Dropsy—Aegle folia, Borabia difusa, Blumia odorata, Berrhaeria ripens, Convallaria, majolis, Lathyrus, Apocynum.

Enlargement of Liver—Azaredicta Indica, Asai, Andersonia, Carduus, Quinia indica, Carica papaya, Chlorodendron infotunata, Kalmegh, Locus aspera.

Epilepsy—Bufo rana, Venanth crocata, Hydrocyanic acid, Veratrum viride, Pas avena, Passiflora inc.

Elephantiasis—Hydrocotyle asiatica, Anacardium.

Enlargement of Spleen—Azaridecta indica, Asai, Andersonia, Ceanothus, Quinia indica, Caryca papaya, Chlorodendron infortunata, Calotropis lectum, Kalmegh, Leucus aspera.

Enlargement of Uterus—Fraxinus americana.

Gall Stones—Biliary Colic—Carduus, Berberis, Hydrastis, Chionanthus, Dioscorea, Cholestrinum, Stignata, Madegus, Perera breve, Thlaspi bursa pestoris, Coccus cactus.

Goitre—Fucus vesiculosus, Iodine, Thyroidine.

Gonorrhoea—Cubeba, Vesicaria com., Cannabis sativa, Colens Aromaticus.

Hydrophobia - Hydrophobin.

Haemorrhagic dysentery—Atista radix, Caster oil, Ciphalandra indica, Ficcus indica, Eupatorium ayapan, Baptisia, Vaccininum metallicum, Aloes.

Haemorrage Cyndon dactylon, Ficcus, Paligioza, Hamamelis, Ferrum phos., Geranium maculatum, Millifolium.

Hysteria—Camphor, Hydrocyanic acid, Pas avena, Passiflora inc.

Hiccough—Kali-brom., Ginseng.

Heart Affections—Crataegus oxy., Cactus grand., Coccus cocti, Makaradhwaj, Aconite nap.

High Blood Pressure—Ranwolfea serpentina, Nux-v.

Insmonia—Passiflora inc.

Insanity—Ranwolfea serpentina, Passiflora inc.

Impotence—Avena sativa, Damiana, Aswagandha, Aeglefolia, Comphor, Cantharis.

Intermittent Fever—Alstonia, Atista indica, Azaredicta indica, Andersonia rohitak, Quinia indica, Chiraita, Chlorodendron infortunata, Cephalandra indica, Calotropis gigentia, Desmadium, Kalmegh, Lencus aspera, Nyctam thes, Olden inandia, Natrum mur bit, Tynosptera cordi-folio, Arsenic alb., Baptisia, Chininum sulph., Eucalyptus glob, Malaria officinalis, Veratrum viride, Cedron, China, Ipecac, Eupatorium.

Jaundice—Carduus marianus, Myrica, Berberis vulgaris, Kala-a zar Asai, Kalmegh, Ceanothus.

Leprosy—Jenocordia odorata, Calotropis, Hydrocotyle asitica, Hygrophilla, Spinosa, Anacardium.

Labour Pains—Caulophyllum, Passiflora inc.

Leucorrhoea—Abroma augusta, Aletris ferinosa, Ova testa, Viburnum op, Viburnum prun., Asoka.

Menstrual Disorders—Asoka, Cimic., Corpus leuteum.

Mental Weakness—Avena sativa, Aswagandha.

Neuralgia—Pas avena, Passiflora, Comp, Passiflora inc.

Nocturnal Emissions—Amalki, Ficcus indica, Hydrocotyle asiatica, Thymol, Bellis parenis.

Nervous Debility—Avena sativa, Damiana, Aswagandha, Alfalfa, Origanum, Mica, Fluid cerefolius, Salix nigra.

Night Blindness—Cod liver oil, Physostigma.

Obesity—Fucus vesiculosis, Phytolire, Aesenbutiner.

Phthisis—Jaborandi, Abrotanum, nux juglans, Natrum pyrodol, Acalypha indica, Ficcus religosa, Blumia odoreta, Hamamelis, Cyndon dactylon, Insticia rubrum. Occimum sanctum, Eupatorium ayapan.

Peurperal fever—Ashoka, Echinacea.

Paralysis—Nux vom, Strychnia phos.

Pits of Pox—Serracenia, Variolinum.

Palpitation of Heart—Avena sat., Crataegus oxy, Blumia odorata, Borrhaevia ripens, Asparagus officinalis.

Rheumatism and Gout—Hymosa, gulthoria, Eupatorium, Belladonna, Urtica urens, Viscum alb. Passiflora inc.

Snake-bite—Leucus aspera, Echinacea. Eupatorium ayapan.

Septicaemia—Fluid calendula, Echinacea, Hemidesmus indica, Hygrophillia, Spinosa, Succus amorga.

Suppression of Urine—Camphor, Coleus Aromaticus, Cyndon dactylone, Fluid cerefolius.

Spermatorrhoea—Avena sativa, Damiana, Aswagandha, Ficcus indica, Makradhwaj, Neufar leuticum, Mica, Saw palmeto, Bellis parenis, Salix nigra.

Suppression of Milk—Recinus.

Senselessness—Amyl nitric., Camphor, Moschus.

Skin Diseases—Calotropis gigentia, Echinacea, Spongia, Cornus alternifolia.

Spasms—Passiflora inc., Passiflora comp., Camphor.

Syphilis—Echinacea, Calotropis gigentia, Cyndon dactylon, Caseara amorga, Hemidesmus indica, Kali iod.

Tremor—Agaricus, Nux-v, Tarentula.

Tumour—Fraxtinus americana, Hydrastis, Condurango, Thuja, Chimaphilla.

Tetanus—Hypericum, Nux-v., Strych., Passiflora compound

Uterine Disorders—Aletris, Farinosa, Hydrastis, Asoka, Janosia, Viburnum op., Viburnum prun.